Strategic Management of Hospitals and Health Care Facilities

C. Carl Pegels, PhD
Professor of Management Science and Systems
School of Management
State University of New York at Buffalo
Buffalo, New York

Kenneth A. Rogers, MBA
Vice President
Planning and Marketing
Millard Fillmore Hospitals
Buffalo, New York

AN ASPEN PUBLICATION®
Aspen Publishers, Inc.   1988

Rockville, Maryland
Royal Tunbridge Wells

Library of Congress Cataloging-in-Publication Data

Pegels, C. Carl.
Strategic planning for hospitals and health care
facilities.

"An Aspen publication."
Includes bibliographies and index.
1. Hospitals—Planning. 2. Health facilities—
Planning. 3. Strategic planning. I. Rogers, Kenneth A.
II. Title. [DNLM: 1. Health Facility Planning.
2. Hospital Administration. 3. Hospital Planning.
WX 150 P376s]
RA971.P4   1988   362.1′1′068   87-19610
ISBN: 0-87189-893-4

Editorial Services: Ruth Bloom

Library of Congress Catalog Card Number: 87-19610
ISBN: 0-87189-893-4

Printed in the United States of America

1 2 3 4 5

Table of Contents

Preface

There are two important reasons why this book on strategic management is important to the hospital/health care corporation manager or administrator and to students of the health care management field. First, the health care industry worldwide, and especially in the United States, is in the midst of a major restructuring. This restructuring process began in the mid-1970s and will continue for at least until the late 1990s. Second, the process and practices of strategic planning have undergone some major changes since the mid-1970s. Whereas strategic planning was practiced by only large corporations 10 years ago, in the late 1980s corporations of every size, including hospitals and health service corporations, must be actively involved in strategic management in order to survive in the increasingly competitive environment.

The major restructuring in the health care service industry is the result of several forces, the most notable being the gradual movement from a fee for service payment system to a prospective payment system. This movement began about the mid-1970s with the provision of governmental support for developing health maintenance organizations and has evolved to mandatory prospective payment systems for Medicare hospital services. Clearly, the prospective payment system will be extended to other third party payers and other settings of health care delivery. Major commercial insurers of health services will increasingly demand that their covered services be reimbursed through a prospective payment system also.

The size and growth rate of the health care industry are other factors leading to its restructuring. Because of its enormous size and its continuing growth rate in excess of population growth and the inflation rate, the health care industry is attracting considerable capital and entrepreneurial interests from outside the traditional health care industry. With this influx of capital and the new entrepreneurial spirit, the level of competition has increased substantially. With increased competition comes necessary change.

All the changes that are occurring in the health care field are not only putting strong pressures on management of the traditional hospitals but also on newly restructured hospitals and the newer health service corporations, such as health maintenance organizations (HMOs), home health care corporations, ambulatory health care centers, nursing homes, psychiatric rehabilitation centers, and substance abuse treatment centers.

The goal of this book is to assist management to deal with the numerous major and minor changes that are occurring in their respective internal and external environments. The book not only provides a structured process for strategic planning, but it also provides many techniques that can be productively utilized in the strategic planning activities of the hospital and health care service organization. Strategic planning in health care is not just an activity engaged in by the president and the senior staff. Rather, it must involve the board of directors and especially the affiliated medical staff. Problems associated in getting these two stakeholder groups actively involved in the planning process are explored and discussed extensively.

Another important contribution of this book is its emphasis on inculcating in the health care manager the need to think in terms of generating and evaluating opportunities not only to remain competitive but also to grow in the face of increasing and threatening competition.

Both authors have extensive experience in health care planning and management. Their perspective is closely related to that of the hospital/health care executive.

Finally, we want to express our gratitude to the Health Administration Press, a Division of the Foundation of the American College of Health Care Executives, for allowing us to use two articles that appeared in *Hospital and Health Services Administration*: "Corporate Cultures and Business Strategy" by Michael O. Bice (Chapter 9) and "Seizing the Competitive Initiative" by Melvin R. Goodes (Chapter 22).

We owe our deep thanks to our dear wives, Patricia Pegels and Kathleen Rogers, for providing moral support during the preparation of this book. We also want to thank Valerie Solly for an outstanding job of typing and proofreading the several versions of the manuscript.

C. Carl Pegels
Kenneth A. Rogers
December 1987

Introduction and Overview

INTRODUCTION

Strategic management is an integrated management activity that identifies where the organization should be heading in the future. The environment in which organizations function is constantly changing, especially so in the hospital and health care industry. As a result, management must constantly be alert to problems it may encounter, threats to which it is exposed, opportunities that it may want to take advantage of, and environmental changes that generate the problems, threats, and opportunities.

Strategic management is a management activity. Although it should be guided by top management and the chief executive should provide leadership, the actual strategic management process should involve all levels of management as participants. In the hospital, of course, the medical staff and the board of trustees should also be involved.

Strategic management is made up of many activities and processes. The first and most important one is strategic thinking, which should guide management's actions at all times and not just when strategic thinking or strategic planning sessions take place. From strategic thinking emerges the strategic plan through the strategic planning process. Strategic thinking also includes the notion of strategic flexibility. Once the strategic plan has been developed strategic implementation can begin. Strategic implementation is frequently identified as a problem area in strategic management. Yet, without implementation a strategic plan is just a document. To ensure that implementation goes smoothly it is imperative that the lower and middle levels of management responsible for implementing the strategic plan take an active part in strategic plan development activities.

These concepts are introduced below, and an overview of the book follows. The reader interested in the detailed discussion of these concepts may want to skip the overview and move directly to Chapter 1.

STRATEGIC MANAGEMENT AND STRATEGIC CHANGE

The leadership provided by the chief executive is an important determinant of the success of strategic management. One of the most important elements of an effective program of strategic change is a partnership between the chief executive and the staff member in charge of coordinating strategic planning. The chief executive provides personal leadership and serves as the catalyst that encourages strategic thinking. The chief planner does the coordinating of the strategic planning activities. He or she needs the full support of the chief executive at all times.

Strategic change requires both top-down and bottom-up participation. Senior management should provide leadership roles, but at the same time must be careful to encourage full participation in the planning process by lower management levels and medical staff.

Strategic thinking should be based on a shared set of values in the organization. There should be a shared point of view about who we are, where are we going, and how will we get there. These shared values or corporate philosophies constitute a set of subtle but powerful levers for strategic change.

The pace and effectiveness of strategic change cannot be judged in quantitative terms. However, Paulson points out that there are useful criteria by which strategic change may be assessed.[1] The following seven factors are important benchmarks by which to evaluate progress in strategic management:

1. Strategies are principally developed by line managers with direct, constructive support by the staff.
2. Real strategic alternatives are openly discussed at all levels within the organization.
3. Corporate priorities are relatively clear to senior management, but permit flexible responses to new opportunities and threats.
4. Corporate resources are allocated based on these priorities and in view of both the organization's future potential and historical performance.
5. The strategic roles of business units are clearly differentiated, as are the performance measures applied to their managers.
6. Realistic responses to likely future events are worked out well in advance.
7. The corporate staff makes contributions of real value to the consideration of strategic issues and receives cooperation from most of the divisions.

These criteria embody a number of issues that need to be resolved before an organization can expect to be successful in strategic management. Organizations that have experienced difficulties with strategic management and especially with the implementation of strategic plans probably will find that they did not meet one or more of the above criteria.

WHY STRATEGIC PLANNING DOES NOT GUARANTEE SUCCESS

Strategic planning as practiced by many large corporations does not always work as well as many claim. Why this is so is explained not so much by the actual planning process as described in this book, but by the way the planning is done and by whom—who are the participants in the planning process.

The whole purpose of strategic planning is to help an organization move from where it is now to where it wants to be at some future point in time. To their chagrin many organizations have found that the process of planning works, but the implementation of the plan leaves much to be desired.

Hayes discusses a few of the reasons for the lack of success of strategic planning.[2] The first reason is that organizations only go through the motions of strategic planning, its rituals, and do not really engage in serious strategic thinking and serious strategic planning that are accompanied by top management commitment. The second reason why strategic planning is not as successful as it could be is because of the top-down orientation of many organizations. To be successful, the strategic planning process must have comprehensive participation by all levels of management, but especially by the lower levels of management that ultimately are responsible for implementation of the strategic plan. Another reason for failure is the development of grandiose strategic leaps, rather than the incremental step-by-step improvements that are difficult for competitors to copy. One of the problems associated with grandiose strategic leaps is that most of the planning of them is done by staff people who most likely will have little involvement with the actual running of whatever operating unit emerges from the grand leap approach. As a result the people involved in implementation of the grand leap probably never were involved in the actual planning and development process.

Therefore strategic planning should avoid grand leaps forward and instead focus on incremental changes and improvements. More important, however, is the imperative to have the participation of lower level management in the strategic planning process. This does not necessarily mean that top management should not actively support and participate in the strategic planning process and give direction and guidance to it. However, it is very important to ensure that there is reasonable participation and consensus among those management levels that will be primarily responsible for the implementation of the strategic plan.

Quinn's study of ten major corporations' processes for achieving significant strategic change also supports the incremental change approach in strategic planning.[3] He discovered that executives managing strategic change in large organizations do not follow highly formalized approaches in long-range planning, goal generation, and strategy formulation. Rather, these executives artfully blend formal analysis, behavioral techniques, and power politics to bring about cohesive, step-by-step movement toward ends that initially are broadly conceived, but that are then constantly refined and reshaped as new information appears. Quinn coined the term "logical incrementalism" to describe the above approach.

One needs to be cautious about devoting too much attention to Quinn's findings. The findings are based on observations of actual processes that may or may not be better than other managerial processes. However, there is considerable support for what Quinn observed; in fact, the Japanese essentially follow similar incremental approaches in their managerial behavior.

One criticism of Quinn's logical incrementalism is that some major leaps forward never would have occurred if everyone always practiced incrementalism. For instance, would the diesel locomotive ever have been developed? Would Boeing ever have developed the 747? Or would new modern steel mills ever have been built? Major leaps have been taken by many firms, and many have managed to do so successfully. As a matter of fact, many firms refusing to take giant leaps—that is, from steam to diesel locomotives—have gone bankrupt.

Therefore, the incrementalism approach to strategic planning is more likely to result in success, but the failure to take great leaps forward where they are necessary can also spell doom for the organization. A sound strategic management approach with full participation by all levels of management will be able to identify when incrementalist approaches and when great leap approaches are appropriate.

In summary then, strategic management cannot just be the domain of chief executives or even top management. It needs to draw on all the skills, knowledge, and wisdom of all levels of management. And management must decide when the incrementalist approach or the grand leap approach is appropriate.

STRATEGIC FLEXIBILITY

Strategic flexibility is the ability of an organization to reposition itself in its market or industry, to enter a new market or industry, to change its game plan, or to dismantle current strategies and adopt a new strategic plan.

Strategic flexibility is especially important for hospitals and health care service organizations because of the current dynamic nature of the industry. A hospital's decision to develop a home health care organization or to acquire a HMO is a major strategic change from the operation of the traditional hospital. Even to consider a major move into a new industry such as the ones stated above requires a strong sense of strategic flexibility.

Strategic flexibility is also an important component of strategic thinking. Too often, organizations engaged in strategic planning tend to think in rather narrow terms about their specific operations within their specific industry and within their specific market. Although this is often commendable, especially in periods of stability, it is dangerous in an industry that is undergoing a massive restructuring process. This does not imply that every hospital should enter other related or nonrelated fields. However, unless opportunities in other areas are explored, little knowledge will be gained and strategic plans may emerge that do not support the maintenance of competitive strength for the organization in the long run.

Harrigan points out that the barriers to strategic flexibility are usually perceived to be asset-specific, but in fact are more likely to be mental.[4] Asset-specific barriers mean that strategic opportunities are viewed to be constrained by the currently available facilities and technological equipment. This view is narrow because of the myopic view of some managers. Another barrier to flexibility is the narrow definition of the product or service in which the firm specializes. For instance, a hospital considers itself an inpatient health care facility but not a health care organization that could provide home health care and outpatient surgical care. A hospital manages a large piece of real estate, the hospital, but does not see itself as a real estate firm. Similarly, a hospital operates an extensive food service operation, but does not see itself as a food caterer. These examples do not suggest that hospitals should enter into any of these areas. However, if the hospital's traditional inpatient market declines, it should certainly consider what its strengths are and how those strengths can be utilized in developing or acquiring other operations that can capitalize on those strengths.

In the past century there have been numerous examples of firms fading away into bankruptcy because they were not flexible enough to react to the technological, social, economic, or structural changes that were occurring in their industry. For instance, the mechanical calculator manufacturer saw his product disappear overnight. The steam locomotive maker faced bankruptcy when diesel locomotives took over.

It is of course not surprising that organizations are reluctant to enter new industries even if they are closely related to their own industry. For one, the entry barrier always exists. However, entry barriers have different levels of height or intensity. For instance, the entry barrier into home health care may be considered to be relatively high because a hospital does not traditionally make house calls and its staff is accustomed to working in one facility. A home health care organization is organized in a different manner than the traditional hospital. However, there are also advantages that the hospital has in the provision of home health care over other organizations with which it will be competing. The hospital is a well-known entity in the community it serves, especially if the market area served by the home health care organization is the same as the market area served by the hospital. As a well-known entity the hospital can utilize its name, which in essence is a brand name and, it is hoped, a well-known and respected brand name. Hence, one can see that entry barriers must be studied and evaluated before a decision is taken to cross that barrier. The important element of strategic flexibility is the evaluation of the entry barrier before a decision is made whether to cross it or not. Without a thorough evaluation of the entry barrier the decision to remain with the status quo—that is, to do nothing—is too easily made.

Strategic flexibility is also concerned with strategic exit or termination. Management of organizations, and this is especially true in health care, have a tendency to hang on too long to a dying operation. If a business unit, such as inpatient care, home health care, or laundry operations, is no longer viable, the decision should be made to abandon it in a timely manner. This is, of course, more difficult in the organization that only has one business, such as a hospital. However, in the future hospitals will increasingly engage in multiple businesses, and the decision to terminate certain businesses when they are no longer viable will have to be made.

In summary, strategic flexibility is a way of strategic thinking that will ensure that management is not myopic. Few organizations have the luxury of operating in stable environments. Health care is functioning in a dynamic environment that will remain so for at least the next decade. In this dynamic environment management must adopt a mode of strategic thinking that incorporates the notion of strategic flexibility as described and illustrated above.

OVERVIEW OF BOOK

The book is divided into seven parts. The first part describes the strategic planning process, including establishing the foundations for the strategic planning process in the organization, specifying the detailed steps required to obtain a well-thought out and well-analyzed strategic plan, and illustrating an application of the strategic planning process. A case study is utilized to illustrate this application.

The second part covers external analysis, including detailed descriptions of three external analysis approaches and techniques for strategic planning: (1) environmental analysis and environmental scanning, (2) industry and competitive analysis, and (3) market research as a strategic planning tool.

In Part III, specific internal analysis approaches are presented and discussed. The first such approach demonstrates strategic business unit analysis versus mission department and service department analysis. Second, financial and operating ratio analysis as a strategic planning tool is described and illustrated. Third, the impact of corporate cultures on business strategy is discussed.

In Part IV matrix analysis techniques are applied to strategic business units. Strategic business units are evaluated and analyzed with the growth share matrix analysis technique and the service area attractiveness-strategic business unit strength matrix analysis technique. An illustration of how the two matrix analysis techniques can be applied to evaluate and analyze strategic business units rounds out this section.

Part V describes matrix analysis for mission departments. First, the application of the growth share matrix analysis technique to mission departments is discussed. Next, mission departments are evaluated and analyzed according to the service segment attractiveness-mission department business strength matrix analysis technique. And last, a case study demonstrates an application of both matrix analysis techniques.

Part VI presents applications of strategic management in three nonhospital health care organizations: (1) ambulatory health care centers including urgent care centers, (2) health maintenance organizations, and (3) home health care organizations.

In Part VII future directions of strategic management are reviewed. First, an extensive discussion and comparison of multihospital and multi-institutional systems are presented. This is followed by a discussion of prospective case payment mechanisms, especially DRGs and their impact on hospital strategies. Finally, the last chapter urges hospital management, in particular, and health care organizations management, in general, to seize the competitive initiative. Health care delivery in the future is going to be an even more highly competitive industry. The successful health care organization in that environment will be the one that best identifies, reacts, and responds to its competition at all levels.

CONCLUSION

Strategic planning has evolved over a period of 15 years from a new managerial activity to a necessity in all major corporations and in many smaller corporations as well. Hospitals and other health-related organizations certainly are not exempt from the need for planning. For a health care organization to remain competitive it must be actively engaged in strategic management activities. It must be able to identify and monitor its weaknesses, strengths, opportunities, and threats and take advantage of opportunities as they arise.

There are many opportunities for strategic management in the health care field as the industry is going through a restructuring process. This restructuring process will force many of the weaker hospitals and other health care organizations out of their current field. Yet, simultaneously it provides many opportunities to stronger organizations, especially hospitals, which, through vertical integration, not only have the potential to strengthen the future of the hospital but also could significantly expand the total size of the new integrated health care organization.

The health care organization that will thrive in the future is either the one that is fully integrated or is part of a larger multi-institutional health care organization. The days are numbered for the survival of single, independent hospitals in the competitive health care market.

In summary, health care organizations must actively pursue strategic management. Strategic management activities as described in this book identify opportunities that will help ensure the continued survival of the organization engaged in the planning activities.

NOTES

1. R. D. Paulson, "The Chief Executive as a Change Agent," *Management Review*, February, 1982, 15–21.

2. R. H. Hayes, "Why Strategic Planning Goes Awry," *New York Times*, April 20, 1986, p. D9.

3. J. B. Quinn, "Managing Strategic Change," *Sloan Management Review* 21, no. 4 (1980): 3–20.

4. K. R. Harrigan, *Strategic Flexibility* (Boston: Lexington Books, 1985, chapter 6).

The Strategic Planning Process

Part I lays the groundwork for the successful development of a long-term strategic plan. It is largely based on personal experiences of the authors in assessing and developing an environment in which useful planning can occur. It reviews the importance of active participation by all parties who have a stake in the successful outcome of the strategic planning process for a hospital. These include the medical staff, the board, upper management, and middle management. To ensure that the planning process is nurtured and the plan is implemented, the full and explicit support of the strategic planning process by the chief executive officer of the organization is critically important.

Chapter 2 identifies and describes the components of the strategic planning process, beginning with the mission statement of the organization and the goals of the strategic plan. Because the time horizon of most health care strategic plans is 3–5 years, the goals stated reflect the 5-year planning horizon. Objectives are developed next. They are based on the goals and are more specific in terms of quantitative measures and time dimensions. Following the determination of objectives the general strategy is developed, which includes tactics—the means of how the objectives are to be achieved. Chapter 2 also presents information on the importance of situational analysis, a detailed description of the firm's current status and condition in terms of revenue, profitability, and competitiveness. Other analysis techniques such as environmental, industrial, competitive, and financial analysis are also discussed.

Chapter 3 is a case study illustrating the various components and processes of the strategic planning process.

Chapter 1

Establishing the Planning Process

HIGHLIGHTS

- Corporate Culture's Effects on Planning
- The Idealization Approach
- Organization Assessment
- The Planning Process and Framework
- Two Main Planning Frameworks
- Creative Participation
- Board Participation in Planning
- Medical Staff Participation in Planning
- Use of a Professional Facilitator in Planning
- Conclusions

1

An organization's commitment to strategic management is best indicated by its commitment to the process of planning. Yet, planning is a most uncomfortable process for many people and is likely to meet great resistance. It takes time away from those day-to-day managerial activities that provide most administrators with the job gratification (and frustration) they seek. Planning forces board members to think actively about the organization's future, which may be difficult. The process of planning establishes the leaders of the organization and reveals the weaker links as well.

In order to avoid the resistance to the planning process and move it into an integral role in the corporate culture, realistic expectations must be set. Good planning processes take years to develop. As long as the commitment to planning remains firm from the top and is integrated into the corporate values system, an effective process that is customized to the organization can be developed. And the better that process, the better the result.

Two different types of planning processes are explored in this chapter: (1) the initial planning cycle, in which the first long-range strategic plan is established and (2) the ongoing process of adjustment and linkage to managerial and medical staff activities. In order to best put these processes in perspective, the organization itself must first be examined for its propensity to engage in planning.

CORPORATE CULTURE'S EFFECTS ON PLANNING

Although the term "corporate culture" has become perhaps an overused term in 1980s management lingo, it is most appropriate in any discussion of the planning process. An in-depth look at corporate culture can be found in Chapter 9. Here it is related to the establishment of strategic management.

A corporate culture most often reflects the personality of the chief executive officer (CEO) and, by default, the top management team that is selected to run the organization. Corporate culture is also often the determining factor as to whether a selected strategy is doable. Waterman discusses a particular organizational model called the "McKinsey 7-S Framework" as a tool for judging the do-ability of strategies.[1] The framework (see Figure 9-2) describes how implementation of strategies is dependent on the organization's unique culture and that a change in strategies cannot easily be carried out effectively without the ability to gather internal support, i.e., move the entire culture. The 7-S framework is a simplified vision of the factors that create the corporate culture and would likewise be considered in any fundamental change that occurs.

The difficulty of moving the corporate culture was described in a 1980 *Business Week* article of some note: "Employees cannot be fooled. They understand the real priorities of the corporation. At the first inconsistency they will become confused, then reluctant to change, and finally intransigent. Consistency in every aspect of corporate culture is essential to success."[2] The article describes the experience of several well-known corporations that had to change management strategies, thereby running up against the impediment of corporate culture. AT&T is probably the best-known example. Deregulation forced the communications giant to move from a customer service orientation to a marketing/sales orientation. The change was drastic, and the corporation's internal struggle with a new identity is legend. The alternative, however, would have been total disaster.

Leadership in developing both a strategic management orientation and an overall corporate culture starts at the top of the organization. It is important to emphasize, however, that the CEO cannot complete this task alone. Hosmer states that it "must be the result of a coordinated group effort, despite the diverse personal interests, behavioral characteristics, group memberships, and hierarchical levels of the members."[3] It is the CEO, acting as the strategic leader, rather than as the general manager, who must integrate and coordinate this effort.

Many health care organizations have been very effective and successful because they are based on a strong corporate culture. Massachusetts General Hospital and the Mayo Clinic are two organizations that come to mind immediately as having a distinct modus operandi and personality. The corporate cultures in these organizations have developed over many years and been nurtured by the leadership and supported by a dedicated middle management/ department head level staff that have identified "the way" of doing things for that organization. The result—organizations have been established that have little trouble recruiting top staff, setting and achieving goals, and maintaining industry leader status. Unfortunately, the complexity of a hospital's organization—especially the differentiation among clinical, managerial, and policy leadership—makes the development of a hospital corporate culture extremely difficult in many instances. Strategic management and a shared vision are key components to making that unique culture a reality. As corporate cultures are usually personality-driven, so too is the propensity for a health care organization to succeed or fail in its planning process. The personality of the CEO is most important because much of the strategic direction of the organization relates to the CEO's personal desire and motivation. In leading hospitals there is also often a clinical leader—that top heart surgeon or other specialist who plays the important role of "hero" to the staff. Get the CEO and the "hero" *committed* to planning, and implementation of the planning process becomes easier. Should either of these players resist, actively or passively, then the planning process will not become a part of the corporate culture.

The leaders of an organization are the glue that keeps the process together. It should never be taken for granted, however, that planning is essentially a group process. In this process, many traditional walls between levels of staff and individuals can come down and representative participation can become a reality. The term "representative participation" is used because a hospital is not a true democracy, and the purpose of representation is to ensure communication between the representative and the employees he or she represents. A reality of any planning process is that employees, clinical staff, and even many board members look to the leaders for guidance on the future direction of the hospital. Representative participation ensures that the plan will not seriously affect the interests of specific hospital family members without the knowledge of their representative. A more specific discussion of interest group participation follows later in this chapter.

Probably the most important concept that is developed in a truly planning-oriented corporate culture is that the idea behind strategic planning—what *should* our business be?—can and should be worked on and decided independently, free of the constraints posed by the thinking—what *is* our business and what *will* it be?[4] One makes the assumption that the business will be different and that change calls for different responses. Any process that can bring the decision makers to that level of thought has made an excellent start.

Establishing a shared vision of the future through a group process is a challenging and often enjoyable process to all who are involved. A great deal of satisfaction can be gained from both leading and participating in the process, because the results are usually obvious and shared by all as a major accomplishment. The main indicator of success, however, is not the written plan, but the shared perception that the organization is moving *toward* a shared future, rather than *from* an existing system.

THE IDEALIZATION APPROACH

A major problem with most planning processes is that the participants limit their visualization skills by taking a retrospective approach. *Retrospective planning* concentrates on identifying and removing deficiencies from past performance of system components. It moves *from* what one does not want, rather than *toward* what one does want. A person who walks toward the future facing the past has no control over where he or she is going. Idealization rotates planners from a retrospective to a prospective posture.

In order to motivate a decision-making group to think positively about the future, it is necessary to use the blank paper approach. This approach quite simply asks planners to create any future they want, as long as it is technologically feasible. All political and financial constraints are removed. Russell Ackoff calls this *idealization*.[5]

This idealization approach has five results, according to Ackoff.

1. It facilitates the direct involvement of a large number of those who participate or hold a stake in the relevant system. No special skills are required; participants can play God. The approach gets people deeply involved.
2. Agreement emerges from antagonistic participants and stakeholders. Idealization is concerned with ends, not means. Awareness of consensus about ends usually brings about subsequent cooperation about means among those who would not otherwise be so inclined.
3. The idealization process forces those engaged in it to formulate explicitly their conception of organizational objectives. It exposes their conception to the examination of others, facilitating progressive reformulation and development of consensus.
4. Idealization forces participants to become conscious of self-imposed constraints and makes it easier to remove them. It also forces reexamination of externally imposed constraints that are usually accepted passively.
5. Finally, idealization reveals that system designs and plans, all the elements of which appear to be unfeasible when considered separately, are either feasible or nearly so when considered as a whole. Planning is oriented to making possible that which appears impossible.

Idealization is by no means a universal approach to planning nor by many accounts the best way to start. Peter Drucker, for one, sees even the best plan as *only* a plan unless it generates into *work*. Every basic management decision is a long-range decision that takes years before it is really effective. That the long-range decision is largely made by short-range decisions is not a conflict here; the process itself is that of moving first toward idealization and then to implementation. Others would see the debate occurring between "soft culture" advocates and "hard number" advocates. Which is more important as an indicator of success—an operating culture or the presence of a comprehensive plan, shared values or natural statistical phenomena? All are essential. Underlying these is the singular concept that, in *any* organization, an environment that stimulates practical creativity in strategic thinking is the absolute requirement for success.

ORGANIZATIONAL ASSESSMENT

The first step in developing a planning process is to assess your organization. Are the right ingredients available to establish planning as a part of the corporate culture? Where are the weak links in the organization for the purpose of planning? What actions must occur before beginning the process itself? Usually, both formal and informal educational activities must occur before the process is begun. These activities focus on what exactly is to be accomplished by the planning process, thereby setting expectations about its time, process, participation, and results. Often a message is passed that the leadership is 100 percent behind the process and will be judging employees on their willingness to participate. More often than not, however, the organization's chosen definition of the planning process is shared, creating a level of expectation and curiosity. However, the expectations should never be set too high, especially in the first year of a planning cycle. Most organizations that have gone through a formal planning process are aware that frustration is a dangerous result because of the inability to link the plan with immediate actions. Figure 1-1 is a schematic diagram of the challenge that linkage brings to the corporate culture. Note the built-in frustration among the members of the strategic planning group when ideas generated usually do not end up either implemented or successful. It is very important to set reasonable expectations.

THE PLANNING PROCESS AND FRAMEWORK

The following section describes the planning process in a way that is understandable from each level of the hospital organization. The corner-

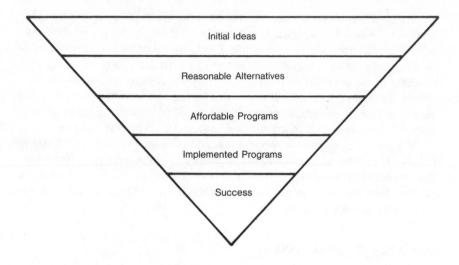

Initial Ideas

Reasonable Alternatives

Affordable Programs

Implemented Programs

Success

Figure 1-1 From Initial Ideas to Success

stones of a successful planning process are consistency and logic. Once the process begins, it must be a continuous closed loop, following a preestablished cycle through management and the board of directors. Participants in the planning process must develop a sense of ownership; the process must not, therefore, revert to a planning department, but must involve those who are most affected by it. A common planning framework must be understood and used throughout the organization. The corporate culture must reward effective planning, and the people engaged in the process must also see its results. In order to accomplish such lofty goals, a shorter-range objective would be to make every employee, physician, and board member a planner. The professional staff planner(s) provides guidance only and assists in developing and implementing the process. Those affected by the plan must have a visible role in putting it together. Once complete, these same people must be fully educated about the overall plan content.

Where does the planning process begin? It begins in the minds of the policy leadership of the organization—the CEO, chairman of the board, and, often, the elected medical staff leadership. These individuals must be fully convinced that only a strategic long-range planning process, adapted to their organization, will forge the controls required to survive and grow. The leadership prepares itself to make the hard decisions that will direct the organization in the long run. They determine the amount of resources of time and dollars that will be expended to establish and maintain the process. They set the goals and objectives for the planning process itself. Through their efforts, a planning framework is established and the end products and time frames determined. Often, the involvement of a planning consultant is valuable because he or she brings an objective set of realistic expectations to the players and helps convince the naysayers that the process really can work for them, too.

TWO MAIN PLANNING FRAMEWORKS

Two main planning frameworks are established before even beginning to plan. The first establishes an initial strategic long-range plan. It sets realistic time frames and processes for accomplishing the first and most difficult long-range plan. The planning cycle for plan initiation is described in Figure 1-2.

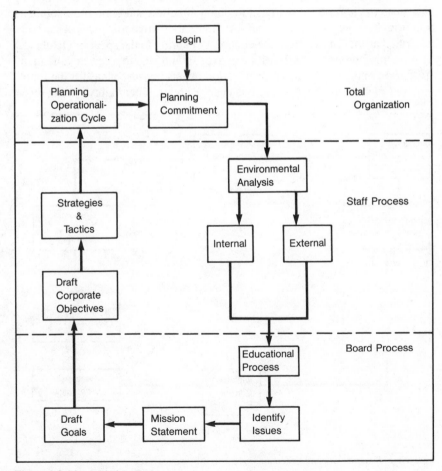

Figure 1-2 Plan Initiation Cycle

The second planning framework deals with operationalization, linkage, review, and update of the planning cycle of the organization. It embodies the true loop concept that incorporates planning into the corporate culture. Figure 1-3 describes this process. The second planning framework is staff-oriented whereas the first planning framework involves the three levels: management, the board, and medical staff leadership. This chapter concentrates on the first framework.

Note that this planning cycle incorporates very specific timing of functions in relation to the budget cycle or resource commitment of the organization. The cycle also links the futuristic, policy-level, long-range plan to the reality of what can be accomplished in a given year. In broad terms, the planning cycle sets the agenda of the organization and provides the resources to move through the agenda. It allows the company to match its resource decisions to chosen strategies and to mesh its top-down direction and bottom-up competition from businesses and resources. At Hallmark Cards, this process has been described as the "move from the euphoria of spring to the spear of October."[6] This ongoing process, if it is truly creative, should lead to a certain amount of frustration in the organization. Frustration results because plans for the future require organization change and this change creates uncertainty among those

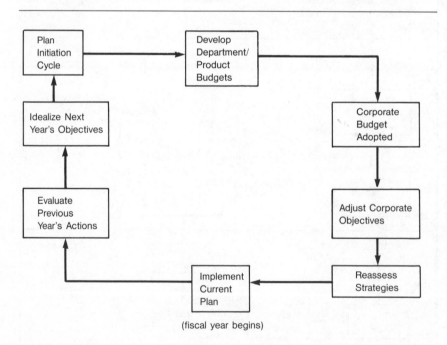

(fiscal year begins)

Figure 1-3 Planning Operationalization Cycle (Staff Process)

affected. If frustration does not result, then the plans may not be sufficiently challenging. A reassessment of your chosen planning process may be in order.

In the process of "planning to plan" the question is often raised about the appropriate time frame for the planning cycle. An ongoing cycle, such as that described previously in Figure 1-3, is based on the organization's fiscal year. However, the long-range plan establishment process is not as straightforward. An easy answer to this question would be to suggest, "whatever feels right for your organization." However, experience tells us to follow several general guidelines in determining the appropriate time frame for the planning cycle.

- Set specific time frame objectives for each step along the way.
- Set specific dates for the Long-Range Planning Committee to assess progress and/or make decisions.
- Always choose a shorter time frame than would at first seem necessary. This forces participants to place priority on the process.
- Never allow more than a year to accomplish the first strategic long-range plan. Enthusiasm will wane, as will the original sense of urgency and purpose.
- Developing the strategic plan in follow-up years should be accomplished in a 2-month period.

CREATIVE PARTICIPATION

Another area of concern, often addressed by consultants, is how to develop creative participation in that first long-range planning process. Ask any CEO of a corporation dedicated to a comprehensive strategic planning process and long-range plan. The most successful will tell you that the key to their accomplishments lies in their ability to back off from the day-to-day operations and look at the "big picture" in the future. Usually this backing off is physical, as well as mental, for example, involving a change of location and method of interpersonal interaction and thinking that may come about at an organizational retreat. Too often we get lulled (or forced) into a rut that is operations driven. Problem solving becomes a short-term objective, rather than a long-term goal. The good CEO cannot afford to stay in this rut very long, nor can a management team be allowed to operationalize itself to death. A decrease in productivity is one of the indicators of the need for a management team to get away to recharge its batteries. Too much to do is just as destructive to productivity as not enough to do. Morale begins to suffer as the managers lose sight of what they are aiming for. The long-term goals may be lost as well when the team does not take the time to relook and re-evaluate.

Backing off or getting away is truly an art, but one that can be taught. It is also a discipline that is best carried out by example. A CEO who is committed to creativity and planning must enforce that commitment by bringing the decision makers into situations where they can concentrate their entire energies on the problem at hand. Note that the term "decision makers" is used here. As a rule, in the corporate world, the decision makers, other than the CEO, are the board of directors. All too often we forget that the board must be brought along in the planning process, as well as the management team. The board members must be active participants in planning for future directions of the organization. Many managers cringe at this very thought. They often ask, "What do board members know about the hospital business that would make them qualified to participate actively in the planning process?" In simple terms, it is not what board members know about health care that makes them invaluable, but it is what they know about hundreds of other endeavors and the simplistic way in which they must approach the health care strategizing session. Board members can be the CEO's greatest ally when they have participated in developing the plan that their institution is following. By looking at the issues from a clearer, less operational perspective, a good board member will be a major asset—someone who is able to pull the management team into the thinking process that becomes inevitably more creative and productive. Can you really explain and justify policies to "naive" board members, or are those policies outmoded or unnecessary and not worth the time to explain?

The "getaway" must be carefully planned to be most productive. It is a general rule that unstructured creative time is not as effective as structured time. For instance, how often have you attended a conference or workshop where the ideas that were raised triggered your thinking about a whole host of issues in your own organization? You race back to your hotel room and write the ideas down and come back to the office all charged up to . . . find everyone else stuck in their uncreative ruts. Frustration is often the result, unless you can excite everyone, but especially the decision makers, about the ideas that excited you in a structured creative moment.

Structuring the organizational creativity to develop long-range goals and strategies is basic to long-term success. The requirements of such a structured creative process include the following:

- An atmosphere for creative development must be fostered through the support and participation of all top management and policy making personnel.

- All persons in the organization must be made aware of the processes by which ideas are managed and the criteria by which they are judged, as well as who the judges are and how to have the ideas heard by the judges.
- The process must be facilitated by a professional who brings the proper participants into the process and provides them with information, instruction, and motivation that will enable them to carry it out effectively.
- A shared data set or information base must be the basis from which all planning proceeds; each participant must draw conclusions from the same set of facts.

Idea generation and creativity can be structured by providing the participants an environment where no outside disturbance inhibits the idea generating activities. This can be accomplished through workshops to provide the participants with sufficient background information followed by retreats to generate the ideas that will eventually produce the strategic plan.

BOARD PARTICIPATION IN PLANNING

One of the mechanisms developed to foster both the creative process and proper participation in planning involves the creation of a long-range planning committee of the board of directors. A word of caution, however, is due here. This long-range planning committee should be a participatory group, representative of the major constituencies of the organization, rather than the board of directors alone. In most voluntary hospitals the composition of the long-range planning committee may look as follows:

- Chairman: Second Vice Chairman of the Board
- Board representatives: former Chairman of the Board, Treasurer of the Board, plus two additional members of the hospital staff
- Administration: Chief Executive Officer, Chief Operating Officer
- Medical staff: President of Medical Staff, Chairman of Medicine, Director of Ambulatory Services, Chief of Cardiac Surgery

The chairman of the board of directors may or may not be a voting member of the committee. Ex-officio status may be granted so that the chairman may participate but not vote at meetings. A board chairman must convey the objectivity and openness of the process to the rest of the Board and may therefore choose to monitor, rather than control it.

Often, hospitals request that employee representatives, especially nursing directors or other clinical staff, have full participation on the long-range planning committee. In publicly held or private for-profit organizations, the planning committee is usually more employee-oriented, with greater control by the CEO and top management. In the more participatory environment of a not-for-profit hospital, the interest groups are more balanced. The board of directors represents the plurality of voting power; their support is crucial in any issue because that group must be responsible for ensuring the proper representation of the plan at the board of directors level.

The CEO of any organization has a major role in the development of a strategic long-range plan. This top employee is retained to provide the policy guidance required by the board. The CEO must look for a balance between overwhelming the committee with professional advice and allowing the process to become disorganized without the necessary control. A good CEO will work closely with the board to educate them, allowing them to reach a consensus on decisions based on information, rather than blind faith. Future support of major decisions will depend on this cooperation.

MEDICAL STAFF PARTICIPATION IN PLANNING

The triangle of power in voluntary hospitals—board, administration, and medical staff—remains entrenched enough in most institutions to require the meaningful participation of the medical staff in the planning process.

It has been argued, in fact, that there is a growing interdependence between hospital boards and medical staffs. This represents a major change since the 1950s when physicians ran the hospital, administration served their needs, and boards were barely visible.[7] Today, unilateral decisions and actions are things of the past. Any move on the part of one party affects the other. Planning is essential to avoid conflict and promote mutual sharing of information. One of the major roadblocks to the inclusion of physicians in the planning process is the differences within the profession itself. Each physician tends to be biased toward his or her own discipline and to put the needs of that specialty above all else. Therefore, it is important to place physicians strategically in multidisciplinary committees, providing a proper balance of opinion.

Because the medical staff must be put in a position to "own" the strategic long-range plan, it must be a major contributor to its development. As with the board of directors, the initial plan development process is an excellent time to educate the medical staff, so that they will become more receptive to the changes that must inevitably occur. Many CEOs and board chairmen have learned the hard way that patience and education are the keys to bringing the medical staff on your side. Proposals and environmental scans must project both the monetary and qualitative changes in medical care practice and must honestly point out the net effect if no change would be made. The hospital that is most successful in establishing a shared vision of the future with its medical staff, board, and employees will have a major edge in successfully completing specific projects down the road.

USE OF A PROFESSIONAL FACILITATOR IN PLANNING

It is very difficult to implement a strategic long-range planning process without a professional facilitator. The planning professional may be on the hospital staff or may be an outside consultant. Many larger organizations establishing their first strategic long-range plans hire a consultant before establishing the staff position in order to determine its job parameters and requirements. Institution of a planning function thus becomes part of the strategic long-range plan itself.

There are many important reasons to hire an outside consultant to facilitate the process. As an objective observer, the consultant is not seen as a threat by any one party involved, and no one is perceived as having a particular influence over anyone else. The resource allocation to a consultant also means that someone on the outside is pressuring the organization to stay on schedule and to produce; the CEO has an ally in this battle for securing management time. A consultant can bring an air of legitimacy to the process, showing examples of other completed plans and how they have affected the organization that hired the facilitator to help them. Experience has shown that doubts about the ability to reach an end in the planning process are significantly reduced when case studies and completed plans are presented. Everyone needs to know where they are headed before they start out.

The role of the consultant must be carefully laid out before he or she is engaged. Expectations, including time frames and end results, must be specific. Ground rules for working with the board of directors and medical staff, as well as the employees, must be laid out to avoid later conflict. A good facilitator is a diplomat, as well as a technician. You are not hiring a person to write your plan for you, but to develop the plan from within the organization. This means that the consultant must be able to draw creativity, information, and personal goals out of people without making enemies, which is a delicate job to say the least. In selecting a consultant, look for enthusiasm, organization, and experience more than any other traits.

The planning professional on a management team is often called on to establish the long-range plan. In fact, many planning professionals are hired for that purpose. This scenario is not necessarily a wise one for many reasons. First, the planner is now a part of the management team, working for the CEO and, therefore, is less likely to disagree with the top leadership. The medical staff may be suspicious of the planner in such a role and be unwilling to come forward with new ideas. The staff planner is not operations-oriented and often thinks differently than the rest of the management team. As the new person on the team, the planner may not receive the respect necessary to establish new ideas, especially because that role does not have to deal with the survival mode that the administration deals in on a daily basis. The staff planner cannot easily work with the board of directors because of the subordinate employee role. Often, the professional planner is put in charge of developing operational plans or certificate of need applications and only does the long-range planning in the available time. For all these reasons and more, a staff planning position should be developed as a result of the planning process and not be created before it is begun.

What is the role of the staff planning specialist? The easy answer is that every organization is different and that planners have very different functions in each hospital situation. However, this response ignores what should be a set of specific guidelines in an effective strategic management framework. The primary role of the staff planner, no matter the title given the position, should be to implement the annual planning cycle. The planner should report directly to the CEO, carrying out the multiyear program necessary to create a planning culture in the hospital. He or she provides support to the administrative staff for linking their objectives and budget requests. He or she assembles, analyzes, and brings information into the decision-making process. The planner typically staffs the board-level planning committee. And, equally important, a system is put in place to manage the bottom-up idea generation process, linking it to the top-down policy and implementation process.

Any planning process must be as inclusive as possible to be effective. The very definition of strategic management is an inclusive, all-encompassing, and ongoing examination of the strategic capacity of the organization. Therefore, it is very important to include in the process those key managers who will be asked to implement the strategic plans. Two of the areas most affected are the human resource and marketing professionals. These are clearly dynamic areas in the organizational hierarchy. Marketing, by definition, is a planning-oriented profession, the effectiveness of which depends heavily on the clarity of the strategic direction of the organization. Too, the human resources professionals will be among the first called upon to implement planning strategies, as most of the moves an organization makes revolve around people. The human resource manager must have a complete understanding of the corporate culture, expectations, and goals in order to carry out successful recruitment and training programs. Including the marketing and human resource managers in the strategic planning process will ultimately lead to far more effective implementation in the future.

SUMMARY

This chapter has provided an overview of the strategic planning process in a large general hospital setting. It identifies the pitfalls and also the opportunities for ensuring full participation of the three power centers in a hospital: the board, the medical staff and the administrative group.

Strategic planning cannot be successful unless it has the full support of the CEO. Ideally, of course, full support should also come from the three power centers of the hospital. The degree of support for strategic planning is also determined by the corporate culture of the organization. The corporate culture must be supportive of strategic planning, and this support must be led by the CEO.

One successful approach to strategic planning is the idealization approach. It requires full participation and support of the top decision makers and must take place in an environment free of distractions.

Two main planning frameworks are introduced and discussed. The two frameworks are complementary and provide guidance to ensure that the planning process does not stretch out over too long a time period. The absolute maximum time for the initial strategic plan should be 1 year.

The importance of both board and medical staff participation should not be overlooked. Implementation of any plan is highly dependent on the extent to which the implementers have been part of the planning process. Therefore, sufficient time should be set aside in the planning schedule to ensure both board and medical staff input in the strategic planning process. The staff planning specialist has a unique role—that of implementing the annual planning cycle through support of the decision maker and the decision-making process.

NOTES

1. T.J. Peters and R.H. Waterman, Jr., *In Search of Excellence.* New York: Harper & Row, 1982, 10.

2. "What Shared Corporate Culture Is and How Shared Values Contribute to the Success or Failure of Strategy," *Business Week,* October 27, 1980, 29.

3. LaRue T. Hosmer, "The Importance of Strategic Leadership," *The Journal of Business Strategy* 3, no. 3 (1982):47–57.

4. Peter F. Drucker, *Management: Tasks, Responsibilities, Practices* (New York: Harper & Row, 1973), 122.

5. Russell L. Ackoff, *Redesigning the Future* (New York: John Wiley & Sons, 1974), 30.

6. Jack Mayer, "Strategic Planning and Marketing at Hallmark," Speech delivered to Buffalo-Niagara chapter of American Marketing Association, April 1985.

7. Raymond C. Ramage, "United We Stand, Divided the Outcome is Less Clear," *Trustee,* September 1983, 19.

Chapter 2

Structure of the Strategic Plan

HIGHLIGHTS

- Planning to Plan
- Describing the Organization
- Defining the Mission
- Defining the Issues
- Identifying, Evaluating, and Selecting Strategies
- Specifying the Goals
- Developing Objectives
- Refining the General Strategy
- Analyzing the External Environment
- Analyzing the Market and Service Segments
- Analyzing the Service Area
- The Internal Environment
- Evaluating Human Resources
- Evaluating Financial Resources
- Evaluating Internal Capabilities
- Summary

2

In Chapter 1 the process by which the strategic planning activity can be established and carried out is discussed. The process itself is most important, and the participants must gain ownership of the plan. This chapter addresses the specifics of the plan itself, identifying its segments and what is involved in putting them together. Much of this chapter is aimed at the professional who has been put in charge of implementing the planning process. By carefully working through each step of the planning process the planner can be assured that no major parts of the plan have been overlooked. Working through each step also helps the planner to assign responsibilities for the various planning activities to other management participants in the strategic planning process.

The steps in strategic planning sometimes follow each other and sometimes must be done simultaneously. Several of the steps must be accomplished repeatedly. Analyses produce information required for moving on to the next step until the plan is complete.

PLANNING TO PLAN

A well-developed and, more importantly, a well-used strategic plan can only be produced by following a reasonably structured planning process. There are just too many different activities and tasks associated with the planning process to do it in an ad hoc fashion. Without structure many aspects of the planning process could be overlooked, and thus an unsatisfactory strategic plan could be produced. An unsatisfactory plan is an unused plan, and an unused plan often destroys the possibility of capturing the decision makers for a second attempt to make a usable plan. In fact, however, even the very best plan—both strategically and in terms of presentation—will be an unused plan unless the decision makers have had a role in its creation.

Thus the process of planning to plan, like a favorite recipe, must be adapted to your tastes and may change somewhat over the years, but the product is good time and again, and the audience looks forward to the end results. Also, everybody does it a little differently, and they all think their way is the best!

The easiest way to illustrate this point is to look at the terminology of planning. Thorough searches of the literature and examination of corporate strategic plans find not one set of definitions and uses of planning terminology but dozens. Military men cringe at the thought of subsuming strategies beneath goals and objectives. Planners argue constantly over whether the goal or the objective is the final destination. The terminology used here has been carefully chosen to reflect the majority of the uses in modern planning. What is most important, however, is not the specific terms used, but *consistency in how you use it in your organization*. It would be wonderful if, as in cooking, a single set of definitions was established, but the planning field is far too underdeveloped to hope for such a standard in the years to come.

The schematic diagram of a suggested planning process is shown in Figure 2-1. The process is somewhat more detailed than that described in Chapter 1. It consists of seven sequential steps or tasks and six parallel tasks that support five of the sequential tasks. The seven sequential tasks are:

1. describing the organization
2. defining the mission
3. defining the issues
4. identifying, evaluating and selecting strategic alternatives
5. specifying the goals
6. developing the objectives
7. refining the general strategy

Six parallel tasks provide input to tasks 2–6. The six parallel tasks are:

1. analyzing the environment
2. analyzing the market and service segments
3. analyzing the service area
4. evaluating human resources
5. evaluating financial resources
6. evaluating internal capabilities

DESCRIBING THE ORGANIZATION

A comprehensive description of the organization for which the strategic plan is being developed must first be prepared. This description is necessary

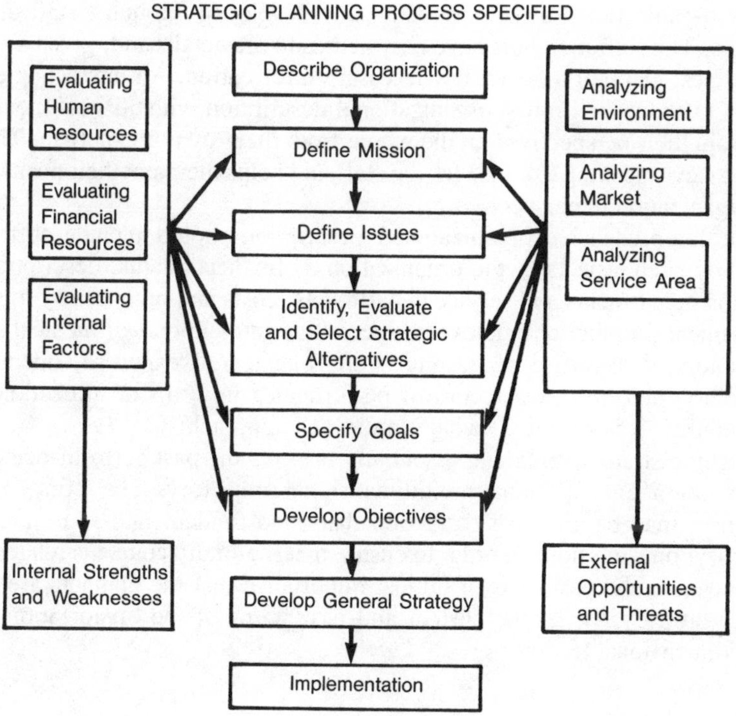

STRATEGIC PLANNING PROCESS SPECIFIED

Figure 2-1 Strategic Planning Process

to ensure that the strategic plan is closely related to the present status of the organization and to ensure that those involved in the process have all the information necessary about the organization. For many decision makers, this is a very interesting and enlightening exercise. All too often, especially in not-for-profit organizations, the board of directors perceives their organization in very rosy or idealistic terms, creating complacency while the organization is in a vulnerable condition. This unrealistic view may be the fault of management (who enjoy their employment and wish to retain it), but often it is a function of the community service or charitable aspect of the hospital that causes it to be seen as a venerable community asset that everyone knows is going to be there forever. Seeing the hard, cold facts, *in understandable terms,* but without judging them, often creates eye-opening reactions that help get the decision makers more involved in the planning process. The organizational description becomes the data base from which the assessment of internal strengths and weaknesses is often made.

The organizational description is usually developed through a staff-driven process. The staff members have easy access to the details and, given a set of guidelines, can pull together the necessary information. An interesting exercise is to share the drafted organizational description with all staff members to obtain their perspectives on the whole from their area of expertise. This is often an eye-opening exercise for the staff and helps them put their position in the organization in perspective.

The comprehensive organizational description should include sufficient detail on such aspects of the organization as financial status, description of mission departments and service departments, costs and revenues by mission department, number of employees, specialties and numbers of medical staff, technological expertise of hospital staff, managerial expertise, operations capability, and historical record of performance in terms of utilization and profitability. It is strictly a "what is and was" approach.

Ongoing strategic planning essentially projects the past performance of an organization onto a future multidimensional trajectory. The "first" plan, however, may be a course correction that is so fundamental as to alter the organization's mission. In order to ensure that the future course is related and connected to the past, it is of utmost importance that the planners are thoroughly aware of what the current and past status of the organization is in multidimensional terms.

DEFINING THE MISSION

If a corporate executive has not suffered through the frustration of wanting to pull away from the day-to-day details and dream about what could be, then it is unlikely that he or she will ever go very far in a chosen field. It is just that tension between day-to-day operations and conceptualization or visualization that drives the top corporate leaders of America. Too much of either the practical or the firefighting mentality may not create the drive that is often the secret of success. Much has been said and written of late about the right side of the brain—that which analyzes and conceptualizes, creates and expounds. That sought-after balance between the practical and the visionary can be learned, but as with every other part of the body, it must be exercised. The corporate body must also exercise its conceptualization powers. One dreamer among linear operations-oriented administrators will find him- or herself shut off and impotent. Likewise, a staff with a dream can be frustrated by a short-sighted board of directors that has not been given the education and/or opportunity to dream with them. The ability and capability to dream and plan for a shared future must be nurtured from the very top to the very bottom of every organization, no matter the size or field of endeavor. The ultimate goal is the sharing of a future, a vision, and the ability to recognize one's own role in that future.

No one statement is more reflective of an institution's ability to conceptualize and project its future than the mission statement. The mission, as a statement of the organizational philosophy and fundamental purpose, should also be a reflection of the personality of the organization and perhaps reveal a little of the corporate culture to its audience. The mission becomes the driving force, the ultimate tool for assessing corporate growth and progress. The mission itself must be tested constantly. Is that dream the current dream? Is the current dream a temporary phenomenon in the overall scheme that has been set out, or is it a real change in direction that must be incorporated into the mission? A mission statement, although not dogmatic, must not be easily changed. There is no higher level of organizational policy change than that which is incorporated into a change or revamping of the mission statement.

Although some professional planners may disagree, it is the authors' firm belief that the goals of an organization cannot be established until after the mission statement is written, at least in its draft form. There are those who would establish goals first and draw up a mission around those goals, but that process ignores the importance of establishing an overall philosophy or tone that serves as a beacon and evaluator of the corporate goals that follow. Those who have gone through the process know that it is much easier to set goals within the guidelines of a mission statement than vice versa. Another cardinal rule of planning is to have the board of directors or chief policy-making body of the organization establish the mission statement and in fact write it when at all possible.

The ultimate success of any mission statement is determined by how well it is known and accepted within the organization. Is the statement regularly discussed and referred to by the policy makers? Are programs and services judged against the mission statement as a part of the prioritization process? Do the employees and their families have easy access to the mission statement and understand its importance to their activities and success? Is management in tune with the mission; do they really believe it or are they giving mere lip service to the philosophy it represents? The mission statement is analogous to the preamble of the U.S. Constitution, and as every schoolchild and new citizen are taught those haunting phrases, so too must the organizational family be able to follow the guideline that the mission sets out.

A good mission statement avoids statistics and extensive description statements about what is. It avoids strategies and tactics, all of which are likely to change. In fact, the best way to judge the quality of a mission statement is to determine the following:

- Is the statement totally understandable by all possible audiences?
- Will the statement be current 5 years from now, assuming that the philosophy of the organization has not changed?
- Does the statement give an overview of the organization so that a stranger will understand it as a whole?
- Is the term "the purpose of this organization is to . . ." used before each sentence? Does it fit?

Exhibit 2-1 shows an actual hospital mission statement. The statement itself was written by the planning committee of the board of directors, from scratch, and edited over a series of seven committee meetings. At each meeting, regardless of what was on the rest of the agenda, another look was given to the mission statement, and inevitably, changes were made. The beauty of the mission statement is that those elements that are most important to the organization are stated at the outset. The hospital's community is defined, as well as its commitment to that community. By writing the mission statement themselves, the board and medical staff are totally committed to it.

A contrasting statement is that of the United Way of America, which in its entirety reads "To increase the organized capacity of people to care for one another." Such a statement could mean that the United Way is a government, a university, the National Guard—you name it. Clearly, such a statement leaves the possibilities too broad!

Exhibit 2-1 Mission Statement

The Hospital Corporation will maintain a leadership position in efficiently providing high quality medical and health care services to the Community. Services will meet identified community needs and shall be provided with concern for our patients and their families. These services will be provided at the lowest possible cost.

The Corporation will sustain and develop educational programming in medicine, nursing, and health-related professions to promote the highest possible standards of medical care and to maintain the availability of appropriate numbers of quality health manpower in the community.

The Corporation will generate sufficient financial resources to meet the operational needs of services provided and to strategically posture for capital needs, technological advancements, and delivery system enhancements.

The Corporation will serve as a responsible employer and participate in the economic and cultural development of the Community.

DEFINING THE ISSUES

One of the major reasons why many strategic plans fail is a lack of focus on issues, especially on those issues that are most crucial to the organization's future. Think of all the specific components of a hospital, for example. Is it possible to address the future of every single area and to put into writing the actions to be taken on every routine operation? Of course not. Yet, many organizations flounder in their planning process because they attempt to be "encyclopedias" of issues, rather than action-oriented documents. By addressing so many issues, it is impossible to address any one issue properly. The plan fails.

The issue-identifying process, therefore, becomes the first prioritization activity. Through staff, board, medical staff, and community inquiries, items of concern are identified and grouped. No attempt is made to develop answers, but only to create categories under which the answers (goals, objectives, strategies) can be developed and structured in a meaningful way. Figure 2-2 shows some simplified issues and their grouping into issue

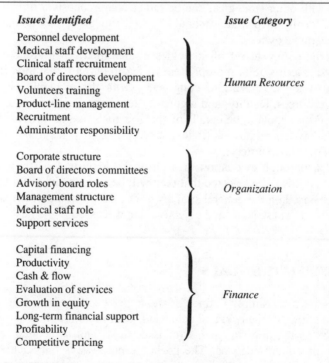

Issues Identified	Issue Category
Personnel development Medical staff development Clinical staff recruitment Board of directors development Volunteers training Product-line management Recruitment Administrator responsibility	*Human Resources*
Corporate structure Board of directors committees Advisory board roles Management structure Medical staff role Support services	*Organization*
Capital financing Productivity Cash & flow Evaluation of services Growth in equity Long-term financial support Profitability Competitive pricing	*Finance*

Figure 2-2 Issue Identification

categories. Issues that should not be part of most strategic plans are such items as plumbing, style of decor, numbers of wheelchairs, and administrator-to-secretary ratios.

Again, the issues chosen are often reflective of the organization itself. The process is one of moving toward a broader understanding, rather than a narrowing vision of how to accomplish the mission. It allows one to see the interrelations of issues before strategies are identified.

IDENTIFYING, EVALUATING, AND SELECTING STRATEGIES

Based on the issues discussed above, strategies need to be identified and evaluated. An identified strategy is determined by a set of goals that need to be achieved. The goals are then derived from the issues discussed in the previous sections.

Each strategy does not necessarily have to be unique. A strategy can overlap with other strategies, can be rather comprehensive, or can be rather specific. Ideally each strategy should be well enough defined so that it can be evaluated on its own.

After the complete set of strategies is identified, each strategy must be evaluated in terms of its appropriateness, feasibility, affordability, fit with the mission of the organization, congruency with the available physical and human resources, legality, and regulatory requirements. Each strategy at this point does not contain the details of specific goals and objectives. However, each strategy should have sufficient specificity so that it can be evaluated in terms of the above criteria.

After a thorough evaluation of each of the identified strategies, a set of strategies needs to be selected that then will become the basis for the general strategy. Based on the general strategy a set of goals and objectives will then be identified. These goals and objectives are discussed in the next section.

SPECIFYING THE GOALS

Goals are most simply defined as the issue-specific aims of the organization that allow for the eventual achievement of the mission. They have been described as mission statements for issue areas and as general, often self-evident directional beacons. The goals are not always fully achievable, although they must be realistic within the environmental context of the plan. They form the outline of the plan and must be in agreement with the mission.

The goals also define the time horizon of the plan. In the 1950s, it may not have been unusual to see a strategic plan with a 10-year time horizon. That was a time of relative structural stability and little environmental change. In today's extremely fast-moving health care environment, a 3-year time horizon is seen as long term, and the need to update on an annual basis is far more crucial.

First-time participants in planning processes often express amazement and sometimes embarrassment at the seemingly too-general or self-evident goals that are produced. The question, "Doesn't everybody know that?", must usually be answered in the negative. What is self-evident to some is new to others. The broader the statement, the easier it is to reach consensus.

As with the mission, the board of directors has ultimate responsibility for the establishment of goals. They are powerful expressions of corporate policy and set the agenda for the institution for years to come. They identify what is important to the corporate culture and provide a specific set of expectations for management and providers alike. Exhibit 2-2 shows the relationship between issues and goals and provides some sample goal statements.

Writing goals is not always an easy task. It is the first opportunity for decision makers to put into writing what they have been merely discussing previously. Issues have to gel and ideas take shape in a consensus-building process. Tensions can build and break as the exact wording and nuances are

---

Exhibit 2-2 Goals

---

1. **Finance**
   1.1 Profitability:
   The Corporation will have operating revenues in excess of operating costs.
   1.2 Competitiveness:
   The Corporation will maintain the ability to compete effectively on a price basis for the group contracts offered by managed care programs.
   1.3 Cash Flow:
   The Corporation will generate sufficient cash flow to meet and exceed corporate requirements.
2. **Organization**
   2.1 Corporate Structure:
   The Corporation will be structured to allow for one corporate Board of Directors with fiduciary responsibility for the entire corporation.
   2.2 Management:
   The Corporation will be structured to provide for corporate management, as well as facility-specific management.
   2.3 Medical Staff:
   The medical staff will be organized as one medical staff with privileges defined on a facility-specific basis.

discussed. Consider an example from Exhibit 2-2. Goal 1.1, profitability, seems straightforward enough on a casual reading, but it could create controversy. First, if this is a not-for-profit institution, the board's setting of a theoretically for-profit goal (not-for-profit does not mean nonprofit) could be educational to its public. More specifically though, it is defining profitability as an operating profit and does not include nonoperating revenues, such as donations and income from investments. Many organizations would find this goal offensive, if not impossible to achieve, because they depend upon nonoperating revenues to make up for operating losses. Goals are not always as simple or self-apparent as they first appear and must be very carefully deliberated by those who are creating the plan.

DEVELOPING THE OBJECTIVES

If goal setting is a policy-making, agenda-building process, then objective setting is a management response of what will be achieved toward those goals in a specific time frame. Often, objectives are stated in the format of a 1-year annual operational plan that responds to a set of goals. However, many organizations include multiyear objectives in their plans as a more specific guide to achieving the stated goals. Whatever the time frame, every goal in the long-range plan should have an associated objective. Often several objectives may be related to a single goal. Objectives are relatively specific, and each has a specific time frame associated with it. Exhibit 2-3 shows specific objectives related to selected goals from Exhibit 2-2.

Objective setting is generally a staff process. Because it involves a specific response and usually is representative of a management style, the objective-setting process must be presented as a staff response to corporate policy. Objectives, being specific, are also the basis for measuring management success in a given year. They should be written in a manner that allows the board of directors to examine progress on any particular goal.

REFINING THE GENERAL STRATEGY

Refinement of the general strategy can be looked upon as a synthesis of the goals and objectives that have been formulated. If goals and objectives are seen as analytical steps and the strategy as the synthesis, then the process of analysis and synthesis, one that is generally viewed as necessary in any thorough planning activity, has been applied.

Exhibit 2-3 Objectives

---

1. **Finance**
1.1 Profitability:
(Goal) The Corporation will have operating revenues in excess of operating costs.
(Objective) 1.1.1 By the end of 1987, operating revenues will exceed operating costs by 10 percent.
(Objective) 1.1.2 By the end of 1987, operating profits will be 20 percent higher than those of 1986.
2. **Organization**
2.1 Corporate Structure:
(Goal) The Corporation will be structured to allow for one corporate Board of Directors with fiduciary responsibility for the entire corporation.
(Objective) 2.1.1 By the end of 1987, the Board of Directors of the subsidiary hospitals will have new bylaws.
(Objective) 2.1.2 By the end of 1987, the Corporate bylaws will reflect the new organizational structure.

However, developing the general strategy is more than just synthesis of the goals and objectives. It embodies an overall strategic outlook for the corporation, which includes the development of relationships among the various functional activities within the organization, as well as development of a relational map among the various business units or market segments of the organization. Functional areas are such areas as marketing, finance, human resources, and operations management. A relational map shows how each business unit or mission department is situated in terms of such factors as business strength, industry attractiveness, market share, and market segment growth rate.

The development of the general strategy therefore provides an overall picture of the organization as it will unfold during the period for which the strategy is developed. By developing the general strategy weaknesses in the previously developed goals and objectives will also be identified.

The general strategy is often stated in terms of functional area plans. For example, the corporate marketing plan should be tied into the strategic goals and objectives, but with a more specific look at an overall strategic direction and tactics for accomplishing the objectives. Strategies can be much more technical and are often seen as the most exciting part of the long-range plan due to their specificity and action orientation. Hospital strategies are usually also formulated for finance (including capital development strategies), human resources development, and medical staff development. Because of its service orientation, however, the marketing plan is most often seen as the key strategy piece in the overall long-range plan.

ANALYZING THE EXTERNAL ENVIRONMENT

Organizations do not exist in isolation. The impact of environmental or external conditions in health care is particularly great at the present time.

A common and usually critical environmental factor is competition, an area that is discussed in detail below. However, there are numerous other environmental factors, such as the effects of government regulations, the economic situation, demographic conditions, technological changes, and social changes.

In essence, an environmental influence can be defined as any factor over which the organization has no control. Environmental factors have been identified as the field and rules under which the game is played. As such, the organization that has the best sense of its environment and that can best use it to advantage will have a clear competitive edge. Planning has been called by some "the cooperative participation with the inevitable." This definition holds true in health care, perhaps more than any other industry. The environment is always changing and creating challenges, leading organizations to review their missions and question their very survival. Change is the key, and the necessity for a decision-making body to be reacting to change constantly will test even the most forward thinking, planning-oriented board.

As with internal issues, countless environmental issues affect the daily operations of a hospital or health care service. The planning challenge is to develop an analytical technique that captures the most important factors of these issues in a manner that helps point to the potential strategies and goals of the organization. One method used successfully is the categorization of environmental issues into "opportunities" and "threats." By this categorization, the decision makers can more easily understand not just the issue but its potential effect as well. Of course, some environmental issues are both threats and opportunities, depending on the strategic reaction of the organization. Often, this type of analysis helps change an ingrained board perception, allowing actions to occur that might have otherwise been seen as undesirable responses to negative environmental factors.

A very important environmental factor in terms of its impact on the health care organization is government regulation. Health care organizations are affected by government regulation of building codes, expansion, operating rules, safety regulations, employment requirements, and of course, reimbursement, especially when the government is the reimburser.

The organization generally can do little to change government regulations and must attempt to function within the constraints imposed by them. In the strategic plan development there must be a constant awareness of current and future government regulations, including possible deregulation.

Environmental projections of future economic situations must be made. How will potential economic changes or government economic policy changes affect the organization? The same question must be asked of changes in demographics, manpower availability, technology, and the social environment. Again, the most important outcome is to provide an understandable analysis that can be digested by the policy makers. Maintain realistic perceptions, as whitewashing of environmental concerns could have major consequences in the future.

ANALYZING THE MARKET AND SERVICE SEGMENTS

In its most basic form, market analysis takes two directions. First is an analysis of the overall market. How much market growth can be expected within the service area in the service segments served by the organization? Second is an analysis of the competitors. How strong are they? Will their numbers increase during the strategic plan horizon? What is the market share of the organization now, and what can be projected in the future in each service segment? Those are some of the questions that need to be answered satisfactorily and completely as part of the market analysis for the health care organization.

Also important in market analysis is a thorough evaluation of the relative competitiveness of each of the service segment niches. Many smaller organizations have been quite successful in concentrating their marketing efforts on relatively small service segment niches. Larger organizations usually concentrate on larger, voluminous service segments. Smaller organizations therefore may find less or, at least, less intensive competition in the small service segments usually referred to as service segment niches.

Relative market share evaluation is also important. If an organization already controls a large market share of a service segment and for that particular service segment there will be little growth, then little growth can be expected for the organization in that particular service segment. By the same token, rapidly growing service segments may provide excellent opportunities, especially for those organizations that have strong expertise in the particular area.

ANALYZING THE SERVICE AREA

Especially for a service corporation, such as a hospital, home health organization, or HMO, the service areas are usually limited by fairly well-defined geographic borders. Beyond those borders services may be difficult to render and are probably not competitive. Therefore, a health care delivery organization must not only define its service area but also analyze in detail all relevant and important aspects of the service area.

Although organizations usually define their overall primary and secondary service areas, they actually have multiple service or product-specific service areas. For instance, the primary service area for inpatient services is the metropolitan area of the city in which the hospital is located. The secondary service area consists of the surrounding area extending for a radius of 25 miles. Similarly, the product-specific service area for emergency room care is different than for open-heart surgery. From a market perspective, it is these more specific areas that carry the greater strategic importance. Certain products can be introduced that affect very targeted markets, yet have little or no impact on the overall service area. Likewise, opportunities for market growth may be in smaller, more specialized niches outside the defined current service area. Therefore, a thorough understanding of product service areas is an important factor in planning success. In marketing language, the service area is the geographic component of a geodemographic market assessment.

Any organization serving the health care sector needs to be fully cognizant of all aspects of its service area. Especially because the health care service area is usually relatively small, the health care service organization is able to become thoroughly familiar with its service area and must do so.

Full knowledge of the service area also allows the health care service organization to project what its needs and the service area's potential will be during the planning horizon spanning over the next several years. In addition, full knowledge of the service area also enables the organization to identify and exploit profitable opportunities, as well as identify potential troublesome areas or threats to the organization during the next several years.

INTERNAL ENVIRONMENT

The internal environment of an organization is that part that can be directly controlled. In a game, it is the players, equipment, training, and coaching. In organizations, it consists of human resources, finances, marketing techniques, selection of services, and infrastructure, among other elements. The corporate culture is part of the internal environment. As with the analysis of the external environment, a framework for internal assessment is needed. The technique most often used is assessment of internal strengths and weaknesses. Specific components are categorized in this manner to enable one to determine the potential for achieving specific objectives. Likewise, strategies are formulated so as to capitalize on strengths and minimize weaknesses.

Three areas of concern to health care organizations—human resources, financial resources, and internal capabilities—are discussed below.

Evaluating Human Resources

In a service industry there is no more important resource than people. Hospitals and health care organizations are among the most complex of human-resource-driven businesses because of the complexities of power structures and technical expertise required to maintain operations. A major component of strategic thinking must be the power-sharing triumvirate in hospitals among physicians, trustees, and management. Each hospital is different in this interaction, with power placed in different proportions in each faction. Of course, other aspects of the human resource puzzle must also be explored and reported. Nursing staffs play an increasingly active part in the decision making process. Technicians abound in hospitals, as do ancillary providers, such as counselors, psychologists, social workers, and therapists. Often overlooked and yet increasingly important are the housekeepers, maintenance personnel, and dietary workers whose work is often judged by clients as most important from a customer satisfaction point of view. Volunteers are often used in a direct service capacity and must therefore be treated as would any employee.

The urge to simplify human resource concerns has been a downfall of many strategic plans. Medical manpower needs must be identified first, as physicians are still the main clients of a hospital. Analysis should include missing or underserved specialties, geographic placement of physician offices, areas with potential community demand for office practices, physician referral (to specialties) patterns, and the age distribution of the medical staff by specialty. Both short- and long-term strengths and weaknesses must be identified.

A major current problem in some areas that will only be increasing in future years is the availability of certain health care professionals. The traditionally low-paying nursing and technology fields will be facing stiff competition in future years as the pool of potential talent shrinks. This should cause more health care organizations to look inward for personnel to fill specific gaps. Hospitals should be doing an inventory of the capabilities of their employees and attempting to reach beyond the barriers of specialization that have restricted job mobility in the health care setting.

To be sure, specialization has many advantages, but an excessive stress on specialization can be counterproductive. Japanese and now many non-Japanese companies as well have begun to downplay the use of the specialized job description. Employees in these companies are encouraged to look at their jobs more broadly while simultaneously retaining responsibility for the specific assigned areas of responsibility. Also more movement within the organization is encouraged, thus giving employees more opportunity for broadening their experience and knowledge of their organization.

The process of performance evaluation, which determines compensation and benefit-plans development, should be addressed. A human-resource-intensive organization must ensure that it obtains maximum effectiveness from its employees. Such effectiveness can be achieved through effective and regular performance evaluations of the employees. The compensation policy should be tied to performance evaluation so that solid contributions by employees can be appropriately rewarded. Similarly, benefit plans should be devised so that the benefits are appreciated by the employees and are seen as a form of compensation over and above their regular monetary compensation.

In order to do all of the above, it is of primary importance that the organization knows of the abilities and interests of its employees. When intra-company openings occur, employees should have the first opportunity to apply for the positions. Although in some cases these transfers may be lateral, they may serve to improve overall morale in the organization.

Another area of assessment must be the formal attempts by the organization to create a service approach to health care through employee orientation and training. It is important at this stage to ask the difficult questions concerning the state of employee morale, the emphasis on effective client relations training, and the support provided through inservice programs to improve morale and quality of services to clients. These are considered investments in the future of any hospital.

Evaluating Financial Resources

The evaluation of financial resources involves more than just determining the financial status of the organization in terms of financial ratios, although financial ratios are an important component of a financial analysis. Financial resources evaluation also includes a detailed assessment of the financial needs of the organization during the planning horizon of the next 3 or more years. Will the organization be able to generate sufficient new capital to finance its strategic plan? Or will it be necessary to generate new capital from external sources? What is the availability of new capital? At what cost will this capital be available? Can the organization afford to add long-term debt? These questions need to be answered in a thorough strategic plan that is preceded or accompanied by a financial resource evaluation.

The evaluation of financial resources should also provide guidance and recommendations to management about the capital structure of the organization. What percentage of total liabilities and equity should be long-term debt? What is an acceptable or desirable current ratio and quick ratio? To what extent can account payables be used to finance operations? What is the accounts receivable ratio, and what can it be expected to be in the future?

Hence, evaluating financial resources is not just restricted to studying the current financial situation in detail but also to trying to project the future and to determining what the future dimensions of the organization's financial structure should be. Needless to say, evaluating an organization's financial resources is a critically important task.

Evaluating Internal Capabilities

Internal capabilities evaluation involves all internal aspects of the organization. Internal aspects of the organization should be analyzed and evaluated to determine how effectively the organization utilizes, applies, or practices in relation to that particular internal factor. However, because human resource, financial, and to some extent marketing factors have already been discussed, the internal factors evaluation can remain limited to those factors not as yet covered.

Specific factors to be evaluated consist of the internal technological abilities, especially in mission departments, such as radiology and laboratory; the marketing expertise; the operations management expertise; the management control practices; the short-term and long-term planning practices; and the ability to control cost. The primary purpose of the detailed analysis of the internal factors is to ensure that the organization is not at a competitive disadvantage vis-a-vis its competitors. Specific questions should be raised as to how the organization compares in relation to the specific internal factor with organizations of similar size in similar service areas. This, of course, is a difficult task and relies on information about the organization that may not always be available. Information on competitors is even less available. However, the best efforts should be used to try to obtain as much information as possible.

In those cases where poor performance on an internal factor is indicated, it behooves the organization to correct its practices. These poor practices should of course be corrected immediately if feasible, or alternatively, correction of the poor practices should become part of the strategic plan. Only by ensuring that every aspect of the organization works at full efficiency and full capacity can one be assured that the organization will be competitive and profitable.

SUMMARY

The importance of structure in the strategic planning process is frequently taken for granted. This is a mistake because there are so many steps to the planning process, and missing one or more of these steps or even certain parts of a step can produce a planning process that is not as thorough as it should be and therefore is a potential long-term liability.

Although the various steps of the strategic planning process are described and charted in a certain order, several steps must be done repeatedly. What is important is that a general process and description of a strategic plan are formulated initially and described by the mission statement. From this general outline can then be developed the goals, objectives, and general strategy.

The steps of analysis can be done independently. Each step must be done thoroughly and probably many times. Thoroughness is particularly critical for the steps of analysis because it is through these that weaknesses can be isolated and strengths and opportunities identified.

Chapter 3

A Case Description of A Hospital: Wheatfield Community Hospital

HIGHLIGHTS

- Organization of Wheatfield Hospital
- Wheatfield Hospital's Financial Status and Projections
- Service Area Description: Demographics
- Patient Population Description
- Medical Staff
- Competition in Service Area
- Comparative Strengths and Weaknesses of Wheatfield Hospital
- Wheatfield Hospital Service As Seen by Medical Staff
- Summary

3

This chapter presents a case description of a hypothetical nonprofit hospital, Wheatfield Community Hospital, which is located in the northern suburbs of a large Midwestern city. The purpose of the case study, which is of a typical community hospital, is to provide a situation to which the reader can apply the techniques, approaches, and processes discussed in this book. The case study describes in detail Wheatfield Hospital's organization and governing structure, financial operations, medical staff, patients, and service area. Also identified are weaknesses and strengths as seen by the medical staff.

Wheatfield Hospital is a full-service hospital with an excellent medical staff. It has 300 beds, and in 1985 it had an occupancy rate of 68 percent. The occupancy rate was rather low, and the hospital administration wanted to increase it, thereby increasing its revenues and surplus so that it could accelerate its repayment program of its relatively heavy debt load. The heavy debt was incurred when a brand new facility was built several years ago to replace a much smaller and inadequate structure.

Management feels that it must increase its medical staff to increase its occupancy rate. However, three of the four hospitals with which Wheatfield Hospital competes are relatively strong; the exception is a smaller hospital. Hence, competition for additions to the medical staff is strong, and it will not be easy for Wheatfield to strengthen its medical staff.

ORGANIZATION OF WHEATFIELD HOSPITAL

As a nonprofit community hospital, Wheatfield Hospital depended extensively on its board, which is comprised of well-respected community members, for its governance. Wheatfield Hospital's current president, Norman Carter, and his predecessor had a good relationship with the board. The board members were able to provide comprehensive oversight of the hospital with-

43

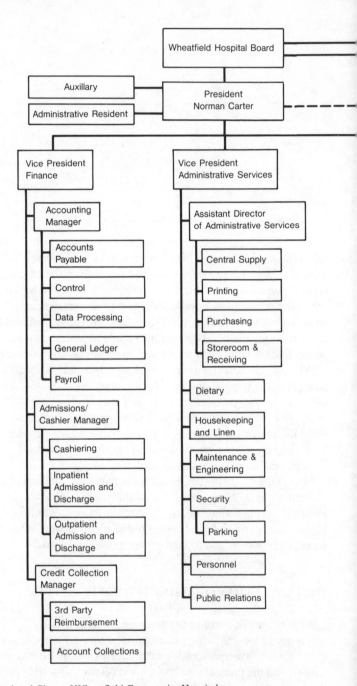

Figure 3-1 Organizational Chart of Wheatfield Community Hospital

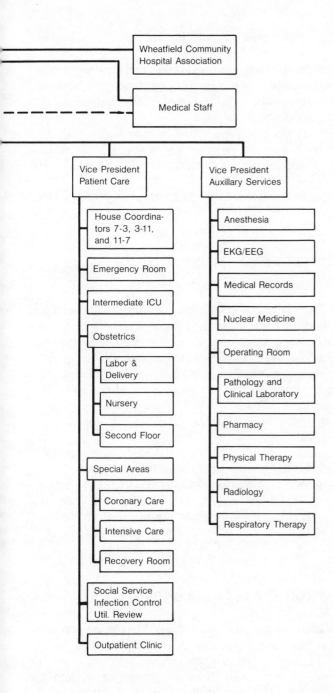

out unduly interfering with management in its daily operations responsibilities.

The hospital's management structure was divided into four divisions; each division was headed by a vice-president who reported directly to Norman Carter, the president. The four divisions were Finance, Administrative Services, Patient Care, and Ancillary Services.

The medical staff had its own organization and communicated with the administration through Mr. Carter on major policy issues. Operationally, each medical staff member had informal communications links at the lower operating levels.

An organization chart, as of December 31, 1985, is shown in Figure 3-1.

WHEATFIELD HOSPITAL'S FINANCIAL STATUS AND PROJECTIONS

Wheatfield Hospital's financial status was reasonable in terms of operations and operating income, as can be seen from the income statement shown in Table 3-1. However, it has an outstanding long-term debt of about $40 million for which it was paying over $3 million in annual interest.

The hefty long-term debt was incurred when the new hospital building was built several years ago. However, so far Wheatfield Hospital had had little difficulty covering its long-term debt principal and interest payments. Its high annual depreciation charge of over $1,250,000 was providing ample funds for sinking fund and principal payments.

In addition to actual financial operating figures for 1985 the vice-president of finance had also developed financial projections for the years 1986, 1987, and 1988. The projections showed increases in net income from $644,000 in 1985, to $800,000 in 1986, $1,430,000 in 1987, and $2,270,000 in 1988.

The real question for Mr. Carter was whether the financial projections could actually be achieved.

SERVICE AREA DESCRIPTION: DEMOGRAPHICS

The service area of Wheatfield Hospital was considered to be the northern two-thirds of the metropolitan area population. Although physicians in the center of the city had affiliations in both the northern and southern suburbs, the overwhelming majority of Wheatfield Hospital's patients came from its defined service area. Exhibit 3-1 provides detailed demographic information on the service area.

Table 3-1 Wheatfield Community Hospital Income Statement of Year Ending December 31

	Actual 1985	Forecasted 1986	1987	1988
Inpatient Revenues	$20,664	$22,300	$23,800	$25,200
Ancillary Service Revenues	3,489	4,105	4,600	5,200
Total Patient Revenues	24,153	26,405	28,400	30,400
Deductions from Patient Revenues	1,481	1,650	1,700	1,800
Net patient Revenues	22,672	24,755	26,700	28,600
Other Operating Revenues	785	810	900	1,000
Total Operating Revenues	23,457	25,565	27,600	29,600
Operating Expenses				
Inpatient Services	13,523	14,797	15,850	16,600
Housekeeping and Plant	1,480	1,670	1,850	2,000
Dietary	1,387	1,750	1,900	2,100
Administration and General	1,957	2,158	2,300	2,400
Total Operating Expenses	18,347	20,375	21,900	23,100
Revenues less Expenses	5,110	5,190	5,700	6,500
Interest on Expenses	3,360	3,300	3,200	3,100
Depreciation	1,285	1,290	1,300	1,400
Net Income from Operations	465	600	1,200	2,000
Interest Income	126	150	150	150
Miscellaneous Income	53	50	80	120
Total Other Income	179	200	230	270
Net Income	644	800	1,430	2,270
Fund Balance—January 1	11,519	12,163	12,963	12,393
Fund Balance—December 31	12,163	12,963	13,393	15,663

PATIENT POPULATION DESCRIPTION

At present Wheatfield Community Hospital serves medical, surgical, obstetrics, gynecological, pediatric, neurosurgery, and orthopedic patients. The distribution of these patients on the basis of admissions is shown on Table 3-2.

In order to increase the census of the hospital it is particularly desirable to increase the number of patients in the specialties of ophthalmology and ear, nose, and throat, and the number of medical/surgical patients admitted by family practitioners and internal medicine specialists.

The census level or occupancy rate during 1985 was 68.3 percent, which was a slight improvement over 1984. However, the hospital administration wanted to see a substantial increase in occupancy in 1986 and beyond. It believed it could achieve a higher occupancy by maintaining the rate of admissions of its present admitting physicians and increase the admissions in ophthalmology and the medical and surgical areas.

Exhibit 3-1 Demographic Description of the Service Area

1. Population	456,000 ('80)	480,000 ('90)
2. Population age distribution (percent of total)		
5 and under	9.8	
6–13	14.2	
14–17	7.6	
18–34	24.8	
35–44	11.9	
45–54	12.0	
55–64	9.3	
65 and above	10.4	
3. Population sex distribution (percent of total)		
Male	47.9	
Female	52.1	
4. Racial mix (percent of total)		
White	82.6	
Nonwhite	17.4	
5. Population income data (percent of total)		
Less than $5,000	16.2	
$5,000–$9,999	22.1	
$10,000–$14,999	29.4	
$15,000–$24,999	18.6	
$25,000 and over	13.7	
6. Reimbursement mix of hospital patients (percent days only)		
Medicaid	16	
Medicare	29	
Private insurance	53	
Self-pay	2	
7. Major employers, number of employees, and insurance coverage		
State University	3600	Metropolitan
Acme Frame Co.	2800	Blue Cross
Ace Trucking Co.	1600	ABC Ins. Co.
Allied Const. Co.	1500	Blue Cross
8. Physicians		
Total number of licensed physicians in service area about 1200		

Exhibit 3-1 continued

9. Trends in service area that will have a positive impact on the hospital next year
   Opening of urgent care center
   Cardiac Care Unit reopening
   Intermediate Care Unit opening
   Increases in outpatient services
   HMO affiliation (ancillary business)
   Closing of military hospital

10. Trends in Service Area that will have a negative impact on the hospital next year
    Unionization
    Overbedded situation in service area
    Continued strong competition

MEDICAL STAFF

Wheatfield Hospital's medical staff is made up of 68 primary care physicians and 38 specialists. Of the medical staff 48 primary care and 25 specialists are major admitters. The physicians who are major admitters are in internal medicine, cardiology, general surgery, neurosurgery, orthopedic surgery, urology, and pulmonary medicine. The majority of admissions to the hospital came from the admitting physicians located in the professional building adjacent to the hospital. A summary of these data is shown in Exhibit 3-2.

During the next year it is anticipated that the major admitting physicians will increase their admissions by 8 percent. In addition, active physician recruiting efforts are anticipated to increase the number of physicians on the active staff by four primary care physicians and five specialists. During 1985 a total of eight physicians were added to the active medical staff, and three physicians were dropped from the active staff.

Table 3-2 Distribution of Patients in Wheatfield Hospital—1985

Specialists	Percentage of Admits
Medical	37
Surgical	17
Obstetrics	10
Gynecological	8
Pediatric	12
Neurosurgery	4
Orthopedics	10
Ophthalmology	2
TOTAL	100

Exhibit 3-2 Summary of Wheatfield Hospital's Medical Staff Status

	Primary Care	Specialists
Number of physicians on active staff	68	38
Number of major admitting physicians	48	25
Number of physicians located in medical building adjacent to hospital	26	18

Current Major Admitting Physicians:
  Internal medicine
  Cardiology
  General surgery
  Neurosurgery
  Urology
  Pulmonary medicine

The types of physicians who will be actively recruited to join Wheatfield Hospital's medical staff during the next several years will be ophthalmologists, ear, nose and throat specialists, pediatricians, and family practitioners.

COMPETITION IN SERVICE AREA

The competition in the service area came from four other hospitals. One of the competing hospitals was smaller than Wheatfield Hospital, and the three others were larger; one of the four was substantially larger. The four hospitals were, in order of size, Pinewood Hospital, Youngstown Hospital, Pendleton Hospital, and Riverside Hospital. The larger hospitals all had higher occupancy rates than Wheatfield Hospital.

The per diem hospital rates were quite similar for all five hospitals. Youngstown had the highest rate at $345 per day and Pinewood the lowest rate at $305 per day. Wheatfield's rate was $330, the same as Riverside Hospital. Except for minor exceptions, all hospitals provided a similar portfolio of services. Table 3-3 shows selective comparative data for the five hospitals.

COMPARATIVE STRENGTHS AND WEAKNESSES OF
WHEATFIELD HOSPITAL

Wheatfield Hospital and its four competitors have certain strengths and weaknesses that explain to a large extent how high each hospital's census is and its ability to attract physicians to its medical staff.

Table 3-3 Comparative Data for Five Competing Hospitals

	Wheatfield	Pinewood	Youngstown	Riverside	Pendleton
Total beds	300	240	350	460	360
Occupancy—1985	68%	58%	85%	74%	82%
Planned additional services	Intermediate care unit	Cardiac care unit	Psychiatric		Ob-Gyn unit
Services Not Offered by Wheatfield		Renal dialysis		Renal dialysis	
Services Offered by Wheatfield only	Neurosurgery				
Semi private rates	$330	$305	$345	$330	$315

Wheatfield's two major strengths are its new facility that was completed just a few years ago and the excellent reputation of its medical staff. However, other hospitals have similar or comparable strengths. The largest hospital, Youngstown Hospital, has an excellent base from which to build its medical staff and thus increase its bed utilization rate. A summary of all strengths and weaknesses is shown on Table 3-4.

WHEATFIELD HOSPITAL SERVICE AS SEEN BY MEDICAL STAFF

A survey of the medical staff revealed some interesting information about how the medical staff physicians viewed Wheatfield Hospital in relation to its competition. A summary of this survey is shown on Table 3-5.

Physicians also made a number of recommendations: that the operating room hours should be expanded to facilitate operating room scheduling, that

Table 3-4 Summary of Strengths and Weaknesses

Hospital	Strengths	Weaknesses
Wheatfield	Excellent medical staff New facility Very good location	Poor community identity Poor referral base for general practitioners
Pinewood	Excellent location	Weak medical staff Appears disorganized
Youngstown	Excellent medical staff	Poor parking facilities
Riverside	Covers all specialties	Weak ancillary personnel High bad debt rate
Pendleton	Strong physician commitment	Poor location Old physical plant

Table 3-5 Wheatfield Hospital's Strongest and Weakest Areas (in Order of Importance)

Wheatfield Hospital's Strongest Areas

Frequent Admitters	Infrequent Admitters
New facility	New facility
Excellent medical staff	Excellent location
Excellent location	Excellent medical staff

Wheatfield Hospital's Weakest Areas

Lack of community identity	Tight operating room schedule
Poor referral base for general practitioners	Preferential treatment for some specialists

marketing efforts be undertaken to improve the hospital's image to the community and to the physicians who are not now on the medical staff.

In response to the question of how the patients viewed the hospital, physicians responded that improved service and friendliness by admission clerks, billing clerks, and nurses would enhance the hospital's image among their patients.

SUMMARY

This chapter provided a case description of a 300-bed nonprofit community hospital. This hospital is currently profitable, has an excellent medical staff, and is located in a growing community. However, the detailed study presented in the case description revealed that Wheatfield Community Hospital has a few weaknesses as well. There was room for improvement in several areas. These areas were identified and could become the focus of the mission and objectives statement.

Part II

General Strategic Planning
Analysis Processes

The three analysis processes presented in this part are environmental analysis, industry and competitive analysis, and financial and operating ratios analysis.

In Chapter 4, environmental analysis addresses the potential effects of demographic, economic, regulatory, political, technological, sociocultural and other changes on the health care industry.

Industry and competitive analysis, which describes the industry in detail and assesses in which direction the industry is heading, is discussed in Chapter 5. Competitive analysis, which frequently is considered a subset of industry analysis provides a detailed scrutiny of the major competitors. This analysis includes an evaluation of competitors' strengths and weaknesses, as well as estimates of their revenues and profitability. The definition of the industry and the identification of competitors are usually restricted to the service area in which the health care organization under investigation functions.

Financial and operating ratio analysis, as described in Chapter 6, is required both for the hospital under study, as well as for the hospital's competitors, provided, of course, that the information is available. The four main financial and operating ratios are liquidity, leverage, profitability, and operating ratios. Also covered in this chapter is a model that determines whether a hospital is financially viable.

Chapter 4

Environmental Analysis and Scanning

HIGHLIGHTS

- Environmental Forces and Impacts
- Critical Environmental Systems
- Regulatory Changes
- Organizational and Operational Changes
- Financial Changes
- Economic Changes
- Technological Changes
- Demographics
- Summary

4

There are hazards in discussing environmental change in the health care industry because it occurs so rapidly and published material can quickly become outdated. Nevertheless, this chapter discusses some basic environmental changes, in simplified form, as examples.

A thorough environmental analysis and environmental scanning process identifies and analyzes environmental influences individually and collectively to determine their current and potential effects on the health care organization. It also identifies potential problems and opportunities. The product of a thorough environmental analysis is a detailed description of the nature of the environments that are critical to the life and vitality of a health care organization.

Survival of a hospital requires that it be able to deal well with an extremely complex and changing environment. Numerous threats exist because of the enormous influence and impact that the environment has on the health care organization. The scanning process allows the organization to remain informed about what is happening or bound to happen in its environment. It is an attempt to reduce the risk of surprises and allow proper marshaling of resources.

ENVIRONMENTAL FORCES AND IMPACTS

Management must constantly be alert for environmental forces that could threaten the current operations it manages. Yet, environmental changes also provide numerous opportunities for profitable expansion or modification of operations. The relationship between environmental forces and planning is shown in Figure 4-1.

In some cases the threats are quickly recognized, and adaptations can be made to avoid their effects. Similarly, opportunities are sometimes seized,

57

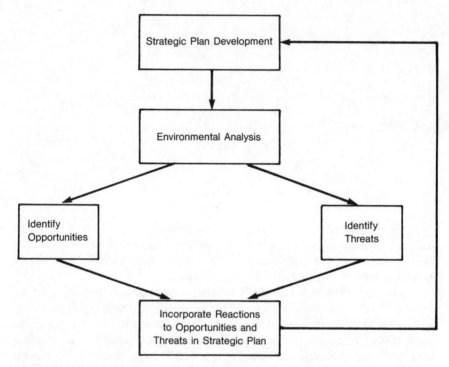

Figure 4-1 Relationship between Environmental Analysis and Strategic Plan Development

but even if nothing is done, a lost opportunity need not always be explained because the perception of the opportunity may not have been pervasive or obvious. Adverse effects of threats, however, can have serious and immediate consequences on operations. Adaptation is not always easy because it frequently means entering a different industry in which the threatened firm has little experience. In addition, required adaptations may require long time horizons, which makes it difficult to react in a timely fashion. Adaptation is a balancing of risks with the goal of the eventual survival of an organization.

In other fields lack of response to environmental changes has destroyed entire industries and many firms in those industries. The railroads' inability to foresee the impact of airlines and to adapt their *missions* to transportation of goods, rather than the limited passenger travel business, caused some of the leading railroad companies in America to close or merge.

Another example of a destroyed industry is the manufacturing of the mechanical calculator. It was replaced by the electronic calculator, which could be produced at only a fraction of the cost. Technology therefore destroyed the mechanical calculator industry. Some firms in the industry managed to adapt to the change. Others could not because the technology of the two products was entirely dissimilar. The more aggressive firms acquired other companies that had the required technology.

Another obsolete product is the reciprocating aircraft engine, which was almost totally replaced by the jet engine in all large engine applications. Again the technology was different, and although adaptation to the new engine occurred because there were no new entrants to supplant the existing limited number of aircraft engine manufacturers, the change was painful. It was even more painful for many airlines who saw their reciprocating engine aircraft depreciate in price quickly on the used airplane market. The only exception was the DC 3, which even today is still in active use.

Environmental changes are not just technological, as the airlines learned when the federal government deregulated the airline industry. Airline deregulation resulted in a proliferation of new airlines and the rapid expansion of some of the smaller airlines. The effect of this capacity expansion was extensive competition, with drastically reduced fares. To be able to compete in this new environment required extremes of adaptation that were not always easy. Those airlines with difficult-to-reduce high labor costs and union contracts were, and are still, facing real difficulties.

The airline industry and the health care industry are analogous in several ways. There is currently a movement toward health care deregulation, which is accompanied by increasing competition and pressure by the largest health care consumers—the government and large corporations—to lower costs. In addition, the organization of health care delivery is rapidly changing. Managed care programs, such as health maintenance organizations and preferred provider organizations, are putting increasing pressure on health care providers to lower costs. The federal government, with its prospective reimbursement system, is putting pressure on both hospitals and physicians to find lower cost alternatives for providing quality care. Price is becoming a factor that threatens the entire traditional base of the health care system. Survival will depend completely on a hospital's abilities to cooperate with the inevitable by using change to its advantage. Those unable to adapt will, like the railroads, be small actors in an industry that has passed them by.

CRITICAL ENVIRONMENTAL SYSTEMS

Environmental analysis is not adequately performed by exhorting management to observe what is going on around them and to take actions accordingly. Environmental analysis is an organized and systematic approach to ensure that any potential environmental impacts will be identified in a timely fashion and to ensure that action is taken accordingly.

To facilitate this environmental analysis it is not only helpful but necessary to divide the analysis into several areas. The environmental areas addressed in this chapter are regulatory, organizational and operational, social, financial, economic, technological, and demographic.

Many regulatory changes now affect the health care delivery organization; their impact will most likely increase in the future. Although there will be increasing deregulation in the areas of pricing, marketing, advertising, and organizational forms, there simultaneously will be increasing regulation in those areas where organizational changes cause or may cause a decline in competition. More than any other factor, regulation is specific to state and local considerations.

Organizational, operational, and structural changes will abound in the health care sector during the next decade. The increasing proliferation of managed care (health maintenance organizations (HMOs), preferred provider organizations (PPOs), national health networks, home health care organizations, freestanding medical centers, surgical centers, and the like) will cause dramatic changes in the ways in which health care is delivered. The numbers of changes are far too complex to begin to address in this book. In addition, they are changing fast enough to make published material quickly out of date.

Social changes will cause the health care consumer to identify more closely with provider organizations than with a single unaffiliated physician. As a result, consumers will identify *their* health care organization with a brand name. This change will be fairly rapid as brand name health care joins the ranks of other consumer products in this country. Product and product-line management is the current trend in reaction to the need for brand name recognition.

Financial changes are extensive in the health care sector. The predominant one is the prospective payment system for hospitals, although the rapid growth in managed care is also significant. These new types of organizations are putting increasing downward pressure on prices in the health care sector. Because they are also relative newcomers in the system, far more sophisticated pricing mechanisms may be seen in the future.

In recent years, business and industry have joined government's call to stem the rapid growth of health care expenditures. Yet, there is some public acceptance of health care taking up an increasing share of the gross national product. The economy as a whole has changed to a predominantly service-driven one. Because health care is part of the service economy, there may well develop an acceptance among the public that it is expensive, but that the expense is a necessary part of the services we have become used to receiving. Public policy response must be closely monitored.

Technological changes have probably been more responsible than any other factor for driving up total health care expenditures. However, as a result of these technological changes, we have diagnostic and therapeutic procedures that are far superior to what was available in the past. Technological changes will continue to have major effects on the health care delivery picture in the future. Of great concern are ethical considerations of deciding who will be the beneficiary of these costly technologies and on what basis will limited resources be distributed.

Demographic change is the last environmental factor that will affect the health care delivery system. The most notable demographic change is the aging of the population. The number of elderly will increase significantly in the future, and their consumption of health care is considerable. Likewise, people are living longer within their high-consumption years. This problem will be increased because there will be fewer younger people to support the older consumers. These demographic changes have both social and financial implications, which will require adaptations in the next 20 years.

REGULATORY CHANGES

Regulation to ensure safe and quality health care will not be compromised while the health care industry is changing. In fact, with the proliferation of different organizational forms of health care delivery, the industry is potentially subject to more regulation in order to ensure quality of care. Regulation will move even further from a focus on cost control factors to an emphasis on quality assurance.

One area where existing regulation will be enforced is the antitrust area. As more and newer forms of health care organizations are established, there will be increasing attempts at mergers, which may inhibit competition. In those cases the Federal Trade Commission will most surely become more active.

However, deregulation is bound to occur in the arena of establishing new health care facilities. Existing legislation will probably be modified to encourage the establishment of more competition. In highly regulated states, such as New York, at least some deregulation will occur in order to foster more competition.

Therefore, the planning body must monitor closely the effects that regulation will have on its organization. In many cases it will pose threats to which management must react. In other cases it will create numerous opportunities for existing organizations to integrate their operations vertically or alternatively to move into entirely new areas, such as preventive care, health promotion, and so forth.

ORGANIZATIONAL AND OPERATIONAL CHANGES

Several major organizational and operational changes are and have been taking place in the health care sector. The most important ones are the rapid growth of managed care programs, the formation of national health care networks, and the move to prospective payment for hospital care. These changes have important implications for all health care providers. Those providers that take advantage of these changes and adjust their mission and operations accordingly will do well. Those health care providers that ignore them will undoubtedly suffer.

Many of the above developments will result in considerably more competition for all providers. HMOs and PPOs will be competing not only with each other but also with other forms of health care delivery. Hospitals, to remain competitive, will have to consider vertical integration seriously. It can be accomplished by affiliating with HMOs, by establishing ambulatory care centers, and by affiliating with or establishing home health care organizations. Similarly, HMOs may want to acquire hospitals so that they can more closely control health care costs in order to remain competitive. Vertical integration, however, must be accomplished while avoiding antitrust act violations.

Far more competition will be experienced in the ambulatory care sector. The solo practitioner will slowly be replaced by the establishment of larger ambulatory care centers and major group practices. These centers will compete against each other but will also be associated with one or more HMOs and PPOs. Solo practitioners will increasingly lose market share to closed panel HMOs and the ambulatory care centers operated by hospitals, health networks, ambulatory care chains, and other provider groups.

Large integrated health care organizations will be the logical outcome of the changes in the ambulatory care sector. These organizations will own and/ or franchise local integrated provider organizations. A typical provider organization may own a HMO, a PPO, a hospital, a number of ambulatory care centers, a home health care organization, and possibly other forms of health care providers. The rationale behind these national integrated providers will be the ability to advertise their services extensively, to provide comprehensive care, to take advantage of a well-known brand name, and to compete effectively on a competitive cost basis. A schematic diagram of an integrated health care organization is shown in Figure 4-2.

Of course, this scenario will not be implemented overnight. However, the logic of the integrated care arrangement is obvious and health care providers should take the above scenario into account when developing their strategic plans.

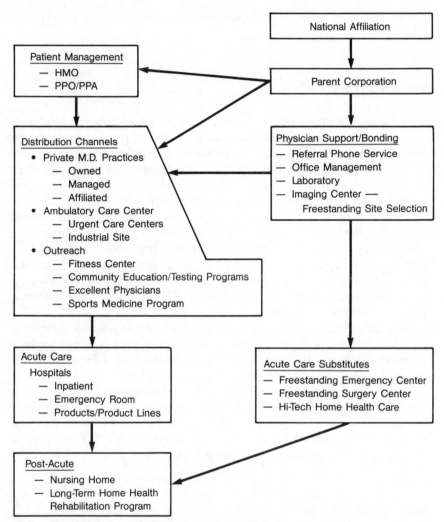

Figure 4-2 Example of Integrated Health Care Organization Components

In addition to vertical integration, hospitals must also be prepared for horizontal integration. Health care organizations, especially ambulatory care centers and hospitals, will increasingly become interested in offering additional services over and above their traditional mix. For instance, the interest in self-care, health education, smoking cessation, exercise programs, and the like will give provider organizations opportunities to expand their operations.

The success of such new ventures depends on basing the creative process on solid market-based data.

FINANCIAL CHANGES

In response to such changes as prospective payment for hospitalization of Medicare patients and the lower charges demanded of providers by managed care programs, management must constantly fine tune its operations.

The reaction of hospital managers to these changes has not been entirely positive. Until recently, hospitals could usually depend on receiving compensation for their services that at least covered their cost. With the new diagnostic related group prepayment systems, cost coverage is no longer ensured. Similarly, volume buyers of hospital services no longer pay at average cost. The service charges are now negotiated and may or may not cover the cost of care. However, aggressive managers have found that, by adjusting their mix of service and gaining control over utilization of their facilities, price competition can be very beneficial. The ability to negotiate for large volumes of patients is a reward for effective cost and quality management.

Financial changes also are affecting HMOs and health insurers. They must be price competitive in order to attain or maintain market share. Setting a price equal to cost or higher is no longer feasible. Prices for services will increasingly be based on competitive conditions.

These changes illustrate the importance to management of keeping up to date with the changes in reimbursement and pricing systems. Because of competitive conditions, management must be prepared to price competitively. For many health care providers this may mean reducing their costs so that they can be competitive with other providers.

ECONOMIC CHANGES

It is interesting to note that, at a time when our economic base is undergoing a massive change from manufacturing to service industries, the concern with rising expenditures in health care is especially acute on the part of business and industry. To some extent the concern about health care expenditures began well before the massive change to a service economy occurred. Fortunately, rate of increase in health care expenditures has moderated, and the concern for rising health care expenditures appears to be abating somewhat.

Another explanation for the reduced concern for rising health care expenditures is the introduction of competition in the health care marketplace. Because of this competition, real or imagined, the general public and public policy makers are no longer as alarmed about increasing costs as they were. As long as the expenditures rise at a rate that is reasonably close to the cost of living then there will likely be little public concern.

In 1986 health care expenditures accounted for about 12 percent of the gross national product (GNP). Many experts believe that this sector will represent probably about 15 percent of the GNP by the year 2000.

Another economic change that will affect the financing of health care is the transfer of payment responsibility from employer to employee. One of the most effective cost-control mechanisms is the cost concern of the careful buyer of health services. Although much of the nation's health insurance premium bill is now paid by employers, responsibility for cost control will shift somewhat to the health care consumer.

TECHNOLOGICAL CHANGES

The inability to recognize or anticipate technological changes can have very expensive consequences for many companies. Environmental analysis, if done thoroughly, will enable the firm to predict and anticipate technological changes so that proper actions can be taken to avoid costly reactions by the organization. Although no single major disruptive technological change has recently occurred in the health sector, it is still necessary for the health care administrator to stay abreast of what is happening in the technological environment.

Examples of technological changes or new technology are new diagnostic equipment, new forms of therapeutic procedures, and new types of drug therapy. Acquisition of new equipment, especially major equipment, is a critical decision for the health care institution. For each major decision on technological acquisition, there is always the question of how soon technological changes will make that new equipment obsolete.

Technology has the potential to improve productivity in many industries. However, in the health care sector technology has usually increased expenditures because of the additional diagnostic and therapeutic procedures made possible by the new technology.

Therefore, health care institutions in environmental analysis must not only look for technological changes that improve productivity but also for those that enable the health care institution to remain competitive in its ability to provide new diagnostics and therapeutics.

DEMOGRAPHICS

One of the great hazards of environmental scanning is the integration of national demographic trends into local planning efforts. Some national trends may not fit into what planners observe at the local level. Therefore national demographic trends are not discussed; instead this chapter presents a practical set of guidelines on what features to look for in a demographic scan.

There is no doubt that, from an environmental standpoint, demographics are the most important and, thankfully, the most accessible and predictable factor in determining health service utilization. The U.S. Bureau of the Census is a source of very sophisticated data that are very pertinent to the health planner. Here are a few rules to keep in mind while thumbing through their countless volumes and computer tapes:

- The Census of Population and Housing is conducted only once every 10 years; by 1989, the 1980 population figures for a community experiencing rapid growth, such as the Sunbelt, will not have a lot of meaning.
- The Bureau of the Census uses both full count and sample data. Read the footnotes and understand the data's limitations.
- The smaller the geographic area, the less accurate the information and the faster it goes out of date.
- Be realistic—planners like to adopt "real" census numbers and are often afraid to comment on their relative accuracy. If your area has many illegal aliens, for example, add on an estimate of their numbers to the official population statistics.

Most localities have a regional planning office with experts on local demographic trends. Use their services as well.

Too often the uninformed amateur health care demographer will point to a major trend—say, an overall population decline of 10 percent—and jump quickly to a conclusion that is otherwise unwarranted. Health care utilization is far more sensitive to trends in population subgroups than to the growth or decline of the population as a whole. In the example above, the 10 percent decrease could be due to an economic downturn, with the decrease being in the healthier working groups primarily; however, the number of the elderly and unemployed—both at risk for health care services—may have increased. Or the decline could be due to lower fertility rates and an aging population, and therefore be the result of fewer children being born. This would have a major impact on pediatric bed need, but may actually result in a stronger demand for adult care. Therefore, carefully dissect the demographic trend into components that are relevant to the health services currently provided or under consideration. Consider the following examples.

- *Age:* In most areas, the fastest-growing population segment is the frail elderly (those over 85 years of age). With life expectancy lengthening, the number of senior adults (65 + years) alone is not a sufficiently sensitive indicator of the type of service that will be needed in the future. A 65-year-old uses very different services than an 80-year-old. Likewise, young children use different services and at a different rate than do adults.
- *Sex:* As hospitals with women's centers have discovered, women use health services in a very different way than do men. Even excluding childbirth, women are still more likely to use health services than men, and almost 40 percent of surgeries performed are in categories affecting only women. Women still live longer than men and have a different likelihood of developing certain chronic diseases.
- *Race:* Although tied closely to socioeconomic factors, there is still a strong indication that race is a predictive factor for utilization of types of health services. In addition, blacks are at higher risk for certain causes of death than are whites and have a shorter life expectancy.
- *Education:* Educational level is a predictive variable that is related both to health service utilization and health status. Prenatal care, for example, is much more likely to be used by more highly educated persons. HMOs have determined that ambulatory mental health services are more in demand by the more highly educated population segment.

Although the above discussion is somewhat simplified, it opens the possibilities that demographic data offer to planning. Because hospitals are moving toward a market-based approach to their service array, it is very important to learn to segment by geographic and demographic subpopulations. For instance, pediatric care delivered by an ambulatory care center provides services to a specific geographic area and within that area to a specific age cohort. Decision makers, especially board members, must be educated to the fine differences and to understand that the geographic target area offers certain demographic opportunities and shuts the door on others.

SUMMARY

Organizations that ignore information about their environment and that do not attempt to predict environmental conditions in the future run the danger of not being prepared when the full effects of environmental changes occur.

Response to an environmental change usually requires considerable lead time, often spanning several years. Therefore, it is absolutely critical that organizations be able to anticipate or predict environmental changes well ahead of the time when their full impact will be felt. With advance knowledge the proper strategic plans can be implemented to ensure that the potential damage of the environmental change can be avoided. Similarly, advance knowledge enables the management of health care organizations to take advantage of the opportunities presented by environmental changes.

Because environmental changes can emanate from many areas management should have a checklist of areas where environmental changes can make an impact. Regulatory, organizational and operational, financial, economic, technological, and demographical changes can all affect your health care institution.

Chapter 5

Industry and Competitive Analysis

HIGHLIGHTS

- Definition of Health Care Industry and Geographic Area
- Competitive Analysis by Rating Mission and Service Departments
- Strength and Weakness Analysis of Competitors
- Competition and Strategy
- Summary

5

It is of utmost importance that a corporation, be it a hospital, HMO, or ambulatory care facility, be fully knowledgeable of the current status, and, ideally, the future status of its competitors.

Clearly, it is impossible to know all the details about a competitor unless you have an informer within the competitive organization. However, in health care it is difficult to have many secrets because hospitals and other health care facilities are relatively open corporations with extensive information flows, especially among professionals who work on a full- or part-time basis in the corporation.

This chapter presents several methods that are useful in evaluating competitors. The first is a rating method of mission and service departments of the competing hospital corporation. The second method lists both weaknesses and strengths of various components of the health care facility. A third, discussed in Chapter 8, is a financial evaluation of each one of your competitors using financial and operating ratios.

DEFINITION OF HEALTH CARE INDUSTRY AND GEOGRAPHIC AREA

Hax and Majluf define an industry as a group of firms offering products or services that are close substitutes for each other.[1] Another important dimension of the definition of an industry, especially for health care, is the boundary of the geographic area that can be served by competing firms. Therefore the term "geographic area" is used to denote the area served by health care units belonging to a single organization.

In the case of a single hospital, a single HMO, or an ambulatory care facility, the geographic area being served—its service area—is reasonably well defined. It is largely determined by the client's travel time and by the

71

accessibility, in terms of availability of public transportation, to the health care facility. Hospitals may also choose to use market share as a variable in determining their primary service area. The farther away a potential patient lives, the less likely he or she is to become a patient, especially if other alternatives are available.

Hence, for a single hospital serving a specific service area, its geographic area and its competitors are clearly defined. Similarly, the location of the existing ambulatory care centers of ambulatory care facilities and closed panel HMOs essentially define their service area and their competitors. If they decide to open ambulatory care centers in adjacent areas, they will of course expand their service area and need to redefine their geographic area and re-evaluate their competition.

For nursing homes the geographic area is more loosely defined. Nursing homes may be able to draw patients from a relatively larger service area than hospitals, ambulatory care centers, home health care organizations, and HMOs. They are usually defined on a regional rather than local basis.

Similarly, open panel HMOs—the independent practitioner association HMOs (IPA-HMO)—are less restricted by geographic boundaries than other health care facilities. The IPA-HMO contracts with solo practitioners or existing group practices to deliver ambulatory care and usually with several hospitals to deliver hospital care. To expand into adjacent areas is therefore quite easy.

For multifacility health care corporations the geographic area boundaries are more loosely defined. Although their boundaries are determined by the facilities they currently operate, acquisition of another facility in an area not being served will, of course, expand their geographic area boundaries. To some extent, therefore, multihospitals, multinursing homes, and multi-HMOs have a much more loosely defined geographic boundary than the single facility health care operations.

Substitute services in the health care sector are limited. If one needs hospitalization there is usually no substitute, except for some elective surgeries. There is, however, a substitute for HMO membership, and that is self-pay or a health insurance plan. Hence, the definition of a geographic area stated at the beginning of this section is quite appropriate for the health sector.

COMPETITIVE ANALYSIS BY RATING MISSION AND SERVICE DEPARTMENTS

The most important activity in industry analysis is the evaluation of competitors in your service area. Because the service area is well defined, competitive analysis is thus restricted to the evaluation of competitors with which a health facility is competing. Of course, potential new competitors must be monitored as well.

There are several ways of evaluating competitors. The first approach is to evaluate the main mission and service departments of a competitor by rating each targeted mission and service department on a scale from 1 to 5. If the department is excellent it is rated as a 5, if it is good it is rated as a 4, if it is average it is rated as a 3, if it is weak it is rated as a 2, and if it is poor it is rated as a 1. Table 5-1 rates three mission departments and three service departments of five competing hospitals (identified as hospitals A, B, C, D, and E) and of the hospital that is doing the competitive analysis, which is identified as AA. Note that only one hospital, hospital C, has a higher total rating (20) than the evaluator's hospital (19). Hospital A has the same total rating as the evaluator's hospital, but the other three hospitals have total ratings lower than the evaluator's hospital.

Not every planner has the knowledge to rate service and mission departments of hospitals in the region being evaluated. Therefore, assistance is required. The best persons to do the rating of mission and service departments are the supervisors of the respective departments in your hospital. They are usually the only ones who will be able to give reasonable evaluations and ratings of their own and their competitor department.

Using a rating scale, such as the one above, always has its pitfalls, and the strategic planner should be aware of the problems associated with it. This scale valued excellent as a 5 and poor as a 1, with increments of 1 between

Table 5-1 Competitive Analysis on Basis of Rated Evaluation of Mission and Service Departments

	Competitors						Evaluator's Hospital
	A	B	C	D	E	Average	AA
MD1	3	2	4	2	4	2.6	4
MD2	4	1	5	1	3	2.8	5
MD3	2	4	3	3	4	3.2	1
SD1	5	1	2	4	2	2.8	2
SD2	1	2	3	1	1	1.6	4
SD3	4	2	3	5	3	3.4	3
Total	19	12	20	16	17	16.4	19

Scale: Excellent = 5
Good   = 4
Average = 3
Weak   = 2
Poor   = 1
Note: MD = mission department
SD = service department

each category. Alternative scales are of course also possible and should be used when deemed appropriate. The 1 to 5 scale is based on the assumptions that (1) weak is twice as good as poor and good is twice as good as weak and (2) improvement from poor to weak is equivalent to an improvement from average to good or from good to excellent. If you agree with the above statements then the 1-to-5 scale is quite appropriate. Remember that the scale selected should reflect how you value the descriptors of excellent, good, average, weak and poor.

The weakness of the above evaluation is that it gives an equal weight to each mission and service department. Such an equal weight is not realistic because certain mission and service departments are clearly more important than other ones. To take the different levels of importance into account, one should use a weighting scheme whereby each mission and each service department is given a relative weight; that is, a weight relative to the other departments being evaluated.

The weighted evaluation method is shown on Table 5-2. Note that the same ratings are used as in the previous example for the six mission and service departments. However, each mission and service department is assigned a weight that is in direct proportion to the overall importance of that department to the hospital. Also note that the sum of the weights is 1.00. By using weights that add up to 1.00, the total average values can be compared more easily.

Table 5-2 Competitor Analysis on Basis of Weighted Ratings for Mission and Service Departments

		Competitors											*Evaluator's Hospital*	
	Weight	*A*	*WA*	*B*	*WB*	*C*	*WC*	*D*	*WD*	*E*	*WE*	*Weighted Average*	*AA*	*WAA*
MD1	.30	3	.90	2	.60	4	1.20	2	.60	2	.60	.78	4	1.20
MD2	.25	4	1.00	1	.25	5	1.25	1	.25	3	.75	.70	5	1.25
MD3	.20	2	.40	4	.80	3	.60	3	.60	4	.80	.64	1	.20
SD1	.10	5	.50	1	.10	2	.20	4	.40	2	.20	.28	2	.20
SD2	.05	1	.05	2	.10	3	.15	1	.05	1	.05	.08	4	.20
SD3	.10	4	.40	2	.20	3	.30	5	.50	3	.30	.34	3	.30
Total	1.00	19	—	12	—	20	—	16	—	15	—	—	19	—
Average	—	3.17	3.25	2.00	2.05	3.33	3.70	2.67	2.40	2.50	2.70	2.82	3.17	3.35

Scale: Excellent = 5
Good = 4
Average = 3
Weak = 2
Poor = 1

Note: W in front of letter indicates that the column values are weighted
MD = mission department
SD = service department

On the basis of the weighted comparisons only one hospital, hospital C, with an average weighted score of 3.70, ranks higher than the evaluator's hospital, hospital AA, which has an average weighted score of 3.35. The four other hospitals have weighted average scores lower than the evaluator's hospital.

Table 5-3 shows the results of evaluating four mission departments in four hospitals with the weighted ratings method. The four mission departments are emergency room, physical therapy, maternity, and x-ray. For the evaluation both a nonweighted and a weighted average were also calculated. The highest ranked hospital on both the nonweighted and weighted basis is Olinda Hospital. The second highest on the nonweighted basis is Camino Hospital, but Marks Hospital is the second highest on the weighted basis. The lowest rated hospital on both the nonweighted and weighted basis is Suburban Hospital.

Assigning weights for the above evaluation method is a subjective decision that should be made by the evaluators. In the last example a higher weight of .35 was assigned to the emergency room, and a low weight of .10 was given to physical therapy. The weight assignments in the example are illustrative and are not intended to be used as suggested weights. Health facility managers usually have a good idea what mission and service departments are more important than others in their respective service areas.

Table 5-3 Competitor Analysis of Four Hospitals

	Weight	Olinda Hospital		Suburban Hospital		Camino Hospital		Marks Hospital		Average	
		S	W	S	W	S	W	S	W	S	W
Emergency Room	.35	5	1.75	4	1.40	3	1.05	4	1.40	4.0	1.40
Physical Therapy	.10	3	.30	2	.20	5	.50	2	.20	3.0	.30
Maternity	.30	4	1.20	1	.30	2	.60	2	.60	2.25	.68
X-Ray	.25	2	.50	3	.75	3	.75	3	.75	2.75	.69
Total	1.00	14	—	10	—	13	—	11	—	12.0	—
Average	—	3.50	3.75	2.50	2.65	3.25	2.90	2.75	2.95	3.00	3.07

Scale: Excellent = 5
Good = 4
Average = 3
Weak = 2
Poor = 1

Note: S = rating from 1 to 5 as indicated by scale
W = weighted rating

STRENGTH AND WEAKNESS ANALYSIS OF COMPETITORS

Another less quantitative, but more qualitative and still very important, way to evaluate your competitors is to examine their strengths and weaknesses. Before examining the hospital as a whole, it is necessary to examine important mission and service departments, departments of medicine, and such factors as location of the hospital.

Table 5-4 is a suggested checklist of the types of strengths and weaknesses that should be identified for six areas of five hospitals. To obtain information on each of the areas will require a considerable amount of intelligence gathering. Once it has been collected it can be kept in a data base and can be updated on a regular basis for use in future strategic planning.

The checklist for developing the strengths and weaknesses file is only intended for illustrative purposes. Hospital or health facility managers must decide for themselves which departments in competitor facilities are important for inclusion in the competitor strengths and weaknesses data base.

COMPETITION AND STRATEGY

In recent years competition has become more relevant to the strategic planner in the strategy formulation process. Porter has identified five forces that govern competition in an industry.[2] Management should consider these forces to ensure that the adverse effects of competition are minimized. Al-

Table 5-4 Checklist for Strengths-Weaknesses Analysis of Competitors

Competitor Strengths	General Surgery	OB/GYN	Pediatrics	Intensive Care	Emergency Room	Location
A						
B						
C						
D						
E						
Competitor Weaknesses						
A						
B						
C						
D						
E						

Note: A, B, C, D and E are designators for competitor hospitals.

though competition is good for the customer because it usually provides better quality products or services at lower prices, it is bad for the producer who must compete. As a rule, the stronger the competition, the lower the profitability.

The five forces identified by Porter as governing competition in an industry are:

1. bargaining power of customers
2. bargaining power of suppliers
3. threat of new entrants
4. threat of substitute products or services
5. jockeying among current competitors

If one or more of these forces is strong, then the profitability of the organization will be affected. Therefore, strategic management should aim to develop strategies that ameliorate these five forces. The more these forces can be ameliorated, the stronger the organization will be in its efforts to improve profitability and overall performance.

Historically, the bargaining power of customers for hospital services has been almost nonexistent. This has changed, however, in recent years with the emergence of HMOs, PPOs, and other new types of health care delivery systems. Customers select HMOs on the basis of economic reasons and also the choice of physicians and hospitals with which the respective HMO is affiliated. Hence, on the basis of force one competition has increased in the hospital industry.

The bargaining power of the critical suppliers to hospitals—the affiliated physicians—has always been strong and will continue to remain so. The increase in bargaining power of customers has not diminished the bargaining power of the physicians.

The threat of new entrants depends on the geographic area in which a hospital is located. In highly regulated states, such as New York, the threat of new entrants is minimal. However, in low regulation states the threat of new entrants is always present. In other industries, such as in the HMO and home health care industries, the threat of new entrants is pervasive.

The threat of new products or services has been particularly severe for hospitals in recent years. The substitution of home health care for inpatient care, the trend toward outpatient surgery in surgical centers, and the emergence of free-standing urgent care centers have been major sources of competition for the traditional hospital.

Finally, jockeying among current competitors to divide up the pie that is left has intensified competition, increased costs, and lowered profitability for many hospitals, HMOs, and home health care organizations.

Therefore management must consider the five competitive forces in strategy formulation. Niches need to be identified in which the threats of competition are manageable. Where the threats exist, strategies need to be developed that aim to ameliorate those threats. For instance, hospitals should nurture their relations with HMOs to ensure an adequate supply of patients. Similarly, active recruiting for physician affiliations should be pursued, especially in those areas where patient loads can be increased. Active lobbying at the state and local level should be practiced by the hospital to keep out new entrants. The threat of competition from substitute services should be ameliorated by the hospital's entry into those new fields. Hospital management should remain continually alert to changes in any of the five competitive forces.

SUMMARY

Industry and competitive analysis of an organization's competitors should be done in a systematic manner. This chapter presented several methods by which this can be accomplished. The first uses both a nonweighted and a weighted rating system of a hospital's mission and service departments. The aggregate and average ratings are then compared with the rating of the hospital that is doing the evaluation.

The second approach lists the strengths and weaknesses of the various components of a hospital. These components can be mission or service departments, but can also include the various departments of medicine, the hospital location, the hospital management staff, and other factors.

The third approach uses Porter's analysis of competitive forces. Potential profitability in an industry is essentially determined by the competitive forces in that industry and the way they affect the organization. Any strategy should therefore aim to ameliorate these forces so as to lessen their impact.

The one area that is not discussed but is important for competitive analysis is a detailed financial analysis of each competitor. Chapter 8 discusses financial and operating ratios of hospitals and other health care facilities.

NOTES

1. A.C. Hax and N.S. Majluf, *Strategic Management* (Englewood Cliffs, N.J.: Prentice Hall, 1984), p. 261.

2. M.E. Porter, "How Competitive Forces Shape Strategy," *Harvard Business Review,* March-April 1979, 137–145.

Chapter 6

Marketing Research As a Strategic Management Tool: Marketing Hospitals to Physicians

6

A marketing department for a health care facility was almost unheard of as recently as the mid-1970s. However, around that time HMOs were being developed. Because marketing prepaid medical care is a major and critically important activity of a HMO, the concept of marketing and market research began to creep into the health care industry.

About the same time hospitals in some parts of the country were beginning to consider and develop marketing and marketing research efforts. However, many of the initial fledgling marketing departments, which were often disguised as "planning departments," were unclear to whom they were going to direct their marketing efforts. Determining the target population was a major problem when hospitals were almost exclusively inpatient-oriented. To be effective, marketing research needs to elicit information on the needs of decision makers. The challenge of hospital marketing is that the decision maker is generally the physician who does the admitting, acting as the patient's agent. Usually, the patient places the hospital decision into the physician's hands, primarily due to lack of expertise and knowledge of alternatives. Although the patient selects a physician, it is the physician who will select the hospital with which he or she is affiliated when hospitalization is required. If the physician is affiliated with several hospitals then the physician will select the most appropriate one or may include the patient in that decision-making process.

Therefore, inpatient hospital marketing and market research activities are primarily directed toward physicians. Marketing in HMOs is both consumer and employer oriented. For nursing homes, ambulatory care centers, urgent

Adapted from *Marketing Hospitals to Physicians—Using Multidimensional Scaling and Hospital Factor Evaluation* by C.C. Pegels and C. Sekar with permission of State University of New York, School of Management, Buffalo, © 1986.

care centers, hospital outpatient centers and emergency rooms, and therapy clinics, the target is more likely to be the patient.

This chapter describes a marketing research study in which the target market was primary care physicians. The survey's aim was to solicit information on what features in a hospital were viewed as critical factors in the physician affiliation decision, allowing the hospital to recruit and retain its primary medical staff more effectively.

MARKETING HOSPITALS TO PHYSICIANS

Formulation of a promotion strategy to increase product or service appeal is based to a large extent on the understanding of consumer or client preferences and attitudes. In fact as pointed out by Green, most product or service market segmentation is based on preferences exhibited by consumers or clients.[1]

The concept of consumer preferences was applied to discovering how physicians choose hospital affiliations for patient admissions and patient referrals. In addition, it was also used in understanding why physicians with multiple hospital affiliations choose certain hospitals more than others for their patients' hospital-related services.

With declining hospital utilization the hospital field is becoming increasingly competitive, especially in communities where the population is relatively stable. Hospitals are difficult entities to market directly to clients or patients because the hospital is usually selected by the patient's physician. To market the hospital it is therefore necessary to convince the admitting or referring physician to use the particular hospital for his or her patients. The physician thus becomes the intermediary between the patient and the hospital. If the physician can be "sold" on affiliating with the hospital and/or using it more intensively, certain benefits would thus accrue to that hospital.

The problem of marketing to physicians is complicated by the fact that many physicians have a set pattern of referrals because of the linkages developed during their practice years. Hospital management thus faces two basic problems:

1. How to increase admissions and referrals from those physicians who are already affiliated with the hospital.
2. How to identify those physicians who will be interested in new affiliation with the hospital and thus be able to generate substantial additional admissions and referrals to the hospital.

Both issues are tied to the attitudes and preferences exhibited by the physicians in choosing a hospital for active affiliation. Actively affiliated physicians are those who actively use the hospital for patient admissions and referrals. Therefore, it becomes important to identify how the physicians perceive the hospitals. Determining the similar and directly competing organizations as perceived by physicians has been achieved by both qualitative analysis[2,3] using judgmental inputs and by quantitative analysis[4] using financial performance as the variable of concern.

PHYSICIAN AFFILIATION PROBLEM

The "best" care for a patient is determined by a large number of medical-related and nonmedical factors. For instance, a study by the authors found that physicians consider such medical-related factors as quality of nursing care, availability of specialists in a reasonable amount of time, availability of state-of-the-art equipment and such nonmedical factors as closeness to their office, attitude of staff and management of the hospital, and availability of parking space as the major factors in deciding on patient admissions and referrals. Because many physicians are actively affiliated with more than one hospital, it becomes absolutely necessary to market the hospital to physicians by highlighting its advantages to the individual physician.

In the hospital that is the subject of this study, called the "study hospital" hereafter, the affiliated physicians already used the hospital a large percentage of time for their admissions and referrals. In other words, the study hospital was already highly regarded by the physicians affiliated with it. Hence, increased utilization had to come from new physicians. Hospital management also decided to focus only on attracting new physicians in the primary care areas—internal medicine, family practice/general practice, and obstetrics/gynecology—because adequate numbers of physicians in other specialties were already affiliated with the study hospital.

Two key questions that needed to be answered for strategy formulation were:

1. What are the demographics and attitudinal characteristics of physicians who will be strong potential candidates for new affiliations with the study hospital?
2. Which other hospitals are directly competing with the study hospital in patient admissions and referrals? On what factors are these hospitals perceived to be similar or dissimilar?

The second question will be answered by an evaluation of the study hospital in relation to competing hospitals and the development of strategies to increase the attractiveness of the study hospital for physicians. Responses to the first question will lead to a focused marketing strategy to attract new physicians for active affiliation.

MULTIDIMENSIONAL SCALING AND HOSPITAL FACTOR EVALUATION

Multidimensional scaling is used for this study to develop groupings of attitudes and perceptions in marketing of products. The technique and application are discussed more thoroughly in Boyd et al.[5] It is also necessary to identify the factors that determine how to group the hospitals on the basis of physicians' perceptions. Finally, it is also useful to develop a portrait of a hypothetical hospital that would be most preferred, i.e., an ideal hospital. Formulation of a competitive strategy is considerably facilitated when answers to the above issues are found.

A two-stage process is used to develop input for a marketing strategy. In the first stage is used a hospital factor evaluation process that elicits physicians' evaluations on a large number of hospital factors that are considered important to physicians. Then in the second stage physicians are asked to make pair-wise comparisons of all hospitals in the domain with which the subject hospital is competing. To these pair-wise comparisons the statistical method of multidimensional scaling is applied. Although each of the above two stages provides considerable information to hospital management by itself, combining the output of the two stages provides a considerable amount of additional information to hospital management for developing a physician marketing strategy.

Hospital Factor Evaluation

Through initial discussions with physicians and hospital management a number of factors were identified that influence physician opinion about hospitals. These factors were then presented in a questionnaire for physicians.

The questionnaire had two parts. In the first part, physicians were asked to evaluate 16 factors that they felt may influence physician affiliation with a hospital. They evaluated the factors on a scale from 1 (extremely important) to 7 (extremely unimportant). In the second part, which listed 19 factors, physicians were asked to evaluate each factor in respect to the particular hospital they utilized most extensively for their patients. The scale ranged from 1 (excellent) to 5 (very poor).

Table 6-1 shows how the physicians ranked the importance of hospital factors in influencing their active affiliation decisions. From this table it is apparent that physicians are very much concerned with (1) quality nursing care, (2) comprehensive testing and diagnostics, (3) pleasant attitude of hospital staff, (4) availability of intensive care, (5) major equipment and facili-

Table 6-1 Factors Influencing Physician Affiliation

		Percentage Response to Factor						
	Mean	1	2	3	4	5	6	7
Quality nursing care	1.552	63.8	25.9	5.2	3.4	—	1.7	—
Comprehensive testing and diagnosis	1.772	41.4	37.9	19.0	—	—	—	—
Pleasant attitude of hospital staff	1.862	36.2	44.8	15.5	3.4	—	—	—
Availability of intensive care	1.862	44.8	32.8	17.2	1.7	3.4	—	—
Major equipment and facilities	1.897	41.4	37.9	13.8	5.2	—	1.7	—
Availability of specialists	1.983	25.9	56.9	12.1	3.4	1.7	—	—
Relations with management	2.483	19.0	36.2	31.0	8.6	1.7	3.4	—
Simpler, quick admission process	2.526	12.1	44.8	29.3	5.2	3.4	3.4	—
Closeness to office	2.825	15.5	25.9	34.5	12.1	5.2	3.4	1.7
Administrative services	2.857	12.1	48.3	29.3	3.4	3.4	—	—
Availability of interns and residents	2.966	19.0	20.7	31.0	13.8	8.6	3.4	3.4
Ease of scheduling surgery	3.019	12.1	31.0	19.0	15.5	1.7	10.3	1.7
Low hospital costs to patients	3.196	12.1	22.4	19.0	32.8	3.4	1.7	5.2
Hospital location	3.328	3.4	22.4	36.2	22.4	6.9	8.6	—
Closeness to residence	3.414	6.9	22.4	25.9	22.4	12.1	10.3	—
Quality of Food	3.690	1.7	12.1	34.5	31.0	10.3	8.6	1.7

Note: 1 = Extremely Important 5 = Moderately Unimportant
2 = Very Important 6 = Not Very Important
3 = Moderately Important 7 = Extremely Unimportant
4 = Somewhat Important

ties, and (6) availability of specialists. The importance of these factors is indicated by their low mean scalar value, as well as by the high percentage of responses in the scalar values of 1 to 3. Of somewhat lesser importance are such factors as (1) relations with management, (2) quick and simple admission process, (3) closeness to office, (4) administrative services, and (5) availability of interns.

Table 6-2 shows how the physicians rated the hospitals they most often use for admissions and referrals in terms of a similar set of factors. This table indicates that (1) availability of specialists, (2) quality of postoperative care, (3) closeness to office, (4) quality of emergency care, and (5) diagnostic services availability are the major hospital factors that determine physicians' admissions and referrals. Most of the other hospital factors are also ranked highly for these hospitals, indicating that in general physicians choose the hospitals that they evaluate highly on most of these hospital factors.

However, it must be noted that Table 6-2 only presents the aggregate summary data for all hospitals used by the physicians. The ratings of individual hospitals provide the discrimination necessary to identify sub-groups of hospitals within the area.

Table 6-2 Hospital Factor Evaluation in Relation to the Most Used Hospitals

| | | Percentage Response is: | | | | |
	Mean	Excellent 1	Very Good 2	OK 3	Not Good 4	Very Poor 5
Availability of specialists	1.707	46.6	37.9	13.8	1.7	—
Quality of post-operative care	1.830	31.0	44.8	15.5	—	—
Closeness to office	1.845	50.0	24.1	20.7	1.7	3.4
Quality of emergency care	1.845	37.9	43.1	15.5	3.4	—
Diagnostic services availability	1.877	29.3	55.2	10.3	3.4	—
Quality nursing	2.052	22.4	53.4	20.7	3.4	—
Security	2.086	25.9	44.8	24.1	5.2	—
MD support services	2.086	25.9	48.3	19.0	5.2	1.7
Availability of equipment	2.103	20.7	53.4	20.7	5.2	—
Ease of scheduling surgery	2.174	12.1	44.8	19.0	3.4	—
Hospital staff attitude	2.246	12.1	53.4	29.3	3.4	—
Adequacy of parking	2.345	29.3	27.6	29.3	6.9	6.9
Hospital neighborhood	2.397	12.1	48.3	27.6	13.8	1.7
Attitude of administration	2.491	12.1	43.1	27.6	13.8	1.7
Availability of interns	2.544	19.0	34.5	19.0	5.2	17.2
Closeness to residence	2.655	20.7	24.1	32.8	13.8	8.6
Administrative systems	2.678	3.4	41.4	36.2	13.8	1.7
Hospital cost to patients	2.759	—	31.0	53.4	8.6	—
Quality of food services	2.810	5.2	24.1	58.6	8.6	3.4

Application of Multidimensional Scaling

The objective of multidimensional scaling is to develop a similarity profile of the hospital being compared. In the domain of competing hospitals in this study there were ten hospitals, including the study hospital. The ten hospitals were then paired up in all possible combinations, producing 45 pairs and for each pair a card was prepared. The physicians were then asked to rank all 45 hospital pairs from very similar to very dissimilar. This was, of course, not an easy task because of the large number (45 in this case) of pairs. It is imperative therefore that the ranking process be broken down in steps to ensure that a valid ranking is achieved.

The process that was developed to rank the 45 hospital pairs is described below. It was supervised by a trained interviewer who provided instructions to the physician as the ranking was performed. The three steps are:

1. Each physician is asked to place the card representing each pair of hospitals being compared in one of five piles marked Very Similar, Similar, Neither Similar nor Dissimilar, Dissimilar, and Very Dissimilar. The physician is asked to keep the number of cards to five each in the very similar and the very dissimilar pile and to ten each each in the similar and dissimilar piles.
2. The physician then sorts each pile from the very dissimilar on top to the very similar on bottom. That is, for the five pairs of hospitals in the very similar pile, he or she identifies which pair is the most similar, which is less similar etc.
3. The interviewer then stacks the five piles in the proper order and assigns a rank of 45 to the topmost card, 44 to the next, and so on until 1 is assigned to the bottom-most card. These ranks are transferred to the similarity ranking matrix in Figure 6-1.

One matrix is obtained for each physician interviewed, and these data form the primary input to the INDSCAL multidimensional scaling computer program.[6]

The determination of the ideal point (ideal hospital) is based on a ranking of all ten hospitals by the physicians. It is obtained with the PREFMAP program which is a statistical computer program that determines the ideal hospital.[7] The ideal hospital of a physician is the most similar to the most preferred hospital and the least similar to the least preferred hospital. Hospital ranking data are collected by asking the physicians to rank the hospitals from 1 to 10 based on which hospital they "most prefer" for active affiliation (rank of 1) to which hospital they "least prefer" for active affiliation (rank of 10).

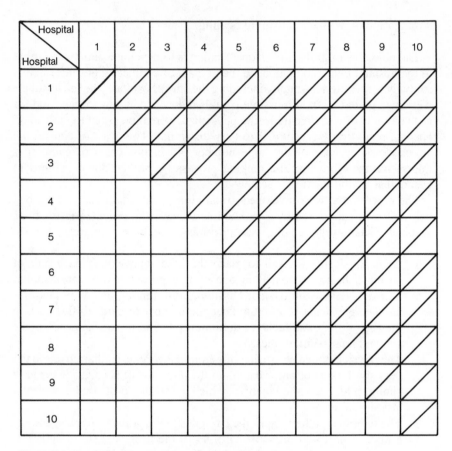

Figure 6-1 Matrix Used for Recording Similarity Profile Ranks

Combining Hospital Factor Evaluation and Multidimensional Scaling

Figure 6-2 presents a two-dimensional plot of the ten hospitals showing how the ten hospitals are clustered or widely separated on the basis of the physicians' paired rankings of them. The multidimensional scaling program is used to locate each hospital on the two-dimensional plot. Next the results of the hospital factor evaluation are used to determine how the two dimensions can be identified.

It can be seen that, across dimension 1, hospitals 1 and 2 are evaluated highly, whereas hospitals 3, 7, 9, 5, 8, and 10 are at the lower end of the scale. Hospital 4, which is the study hospital, is evaluated satisfactorily on this dimension. Similarly, on dimension 2 hospitals 3, 7, 9, 4, and 2 are

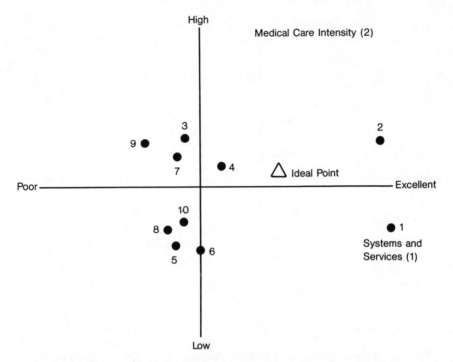

Figure 6-2 Physician Perceptions of Hospitals: Aggregate Analysis, Dimensions 1 and 2

viewed positively, and the other hospitals are considered weak. It is important to note that the positioning on the dimensions is relative; that is, negative
values do not indicate negative evaluation of the hospital, but indicate that
these hospitals are considered relatively lower on that dimension compared to
others.

Based on the analysis of the hospital factors considered important and the
evaluation of individual hospitals compared to the average evaluation, it was
determined that dimension 1 should be identified as MD Support Services/
Admission and Discharge Systems, because it discriminates hospitals 1 and 2
from hospitals 3, 5, 6, 7, 8, 9, and 10. Similarly, dimension 2 should be
identified as Quick Availability of Specialists/Emergency Care Services. Or
dimension 1 could be called Systems and Services and dimension 2 could be
identified as Medical Care Intensity.

In this case the multidimensional scaling allows the use of a third dimension that is shown to be statistically significant. Figure 6-3 shows the same
hospitals in dimensions 1 and 3. Along dimension 3, hospitals 3, 4, 5, 6, 7,
and 8 as a group are considered better than two smaller groups of hospitals

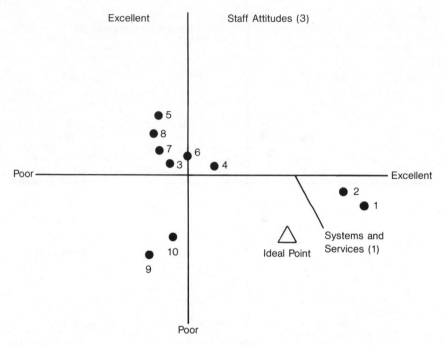

Figure 6-3 Physician Perceptions of Hospitals: Aggregate Analysis, Dimensions 1 and 3

consisting of hospitals 9 and 10 and hospitals 1 and 2. The major reasons for the above differences seem to be the attitude of management and the attitude of the hospital staff. This dimension is therefore referred to as Attitude.

Based on these three dimensions the following groups of hospitals emerge:

- *Group 1: The Best*—Hospital 2: Good on systems and services and patient care; somewhat deficient on attitudes
- *Group 2: The Average*—Hospital 4: OK on all dimensions, but not significantly high on any dimension
- *Group 3: The Functionalist*—Hospital 1: Good on systems and services, but low on patient care and attitudes
- *Group 4: The Bureaucratic*—Hospital 3 and 7: Weak on system and services, but good on patient care and attitudes
- *Group 5: The Poor Performers*—Hospitals 5, 6, 7, 8, 9, and 10: Weak on at least two of the three dimensions.

It is clear that hospital 4, the focus of our study, has to prove its attractiveness compared to Group 1 and Group 3 hospitals. Although it is possible to attract some physicians from other hospitals, the study clearly indicates that improvements in the three dimensions by the study hospital will improve its attractiveness. Furthermore, the physicians who use hospitals 1 and 2 consider hospital 4 as a possible alternative because of the location and similarities in terms of medical care and quality. The location of the ideal point (the ideal hospital) also reveals that hospital 4 should be moving toward hospitals 1 and 2. It should be noted that the ideal hospital described here is based on the preferences among the available choices and is not an absolute ideal.

SUMMARY

Based on the above results, management of the study hospital can now begin to formulate appropriate strategies to attract physicians who are currently affiliated with other hospitals. A reasonable marketing strategy would be one that stresses the hospital factors found to be important to the physicians.

The detailed analysis described in the chapter led to the identification of a group of physicians who are potential targets for affiliation with the study hospital. Whether the study hospital will be successful in attracting the targeted physicians is as yet unknown.

This chapter has shown how a multidimensional scaling technique, often used by consumer product marketers, together with an extensive hospital factor survey, can be used to develop a marketing plan for a complex entity, such as a hospital. Administering the multidimensional scaling instrument is a necessary part of the process but one that could be quite tedious unless appropriate steps are followed. Specific marketing strategies can be developed based on the results of the analysis.

NOTES

1. Paul E. Green, "Marketing Applications of MDs: Assessment and Outlook," *Journal of Marketing*, 39 (1975):24–31.

2. Michael E. Porter, *Competitive Strategy: Techniques for Analyzing Industries and Competitors* (New York: Free Press, 1980), chapters 3–5.

3. William E. Rothschild, *How to Gain (and Maintain) The Competitive Advantage in Business* (New York: McGraw Hill, 1984), chapters 3–7.

4. Kenneth J. Hatten, "Strategic Models in the Brewing Industry," Ph.D. Diss. Purdue University, 1974, 19–47.

5. Harper W. Boyd, Ralph Westfall, and Stash F. Stanley, *Marketing Research: Texts and Cases* (Richard Irwin, 1981), chapters 3–5.

6. John D. Carroll and John J. Chang, "INDSCAL-S: Program for Individual Differences and Multidimensional Scaling," Morristown, N.J.: Bell Communications Research, 1974.

7. John D. Carroll and John J. Chang, "Multidimensional Scaling via a Generalization of Coombs' Unfolding Model," Morristown, N.J.: Bell Communications Research, 1973.

Part III

Special Strategic Management Analysis Processes

Chapter 7 describes and defines the strategic business unit, the mission department and the service department. The strategic business unit (SBU) is a common concept in strategic management and largely applies to multi-institutional health care organizations in the health care field. The mission department and the service department are commonly accepted concepts in the single hospital or in other health care settings. Having clear definitions for each is an important prerequisite for strategic management.

Marketing research as a strategic management tool is reviewed in Chapter 8. Marketing for a hospital must always include means and methods to obtain or retain affiliated physicians who admit patients to the hospital or refer patients for specialized procedures. A marketing research process is illustrated that enables management to identify what kind of marketing strategy it should pursue in order to attract new physicians and retain existing physicians.

The issue of corporate cultures and strategic plan development is addressed in Chapter 9. The study of corporate cultures has increased considerably since its importance became evident in the late 1970s. It was found then that in Japan positive corporate cultures seemed to have a considerable positive influence on the performance of companies. It has since been found that corporate cultures differ significantly among organizations and that some American companies also have highly positive corporate cultures. It was also discovered that it is extremely difficult, costly, and time consuming to change the corporate culture in an organization. Therefore, assessing what the status of the corporate culture is in an organization is an important part of the strategic management process.

Chapter 7

Strategic Business Unit versus Mission and Service Department Planning

HIGHLIGHTS

- Description of a Strategic Business Unit (SBU)
- Definitions of a Mission Department (MD) and a Service Department (SD)
- Definition of Mission and Service Department Sectors in Corporate Planning
- Corporate Strategic Planning for Health Facilities
- Generic Strategies for Corporate Planning
- Vertical Integration
- Horizontal Integration
- Corporate Reorganization
- Summary

There are three levels at which strategic planning should take place in the large health care corporation. These three levels are the corporate level, the strategic business unit (SBU) level, and the mission and service department level, as shown on Figure 7-1.

Not only should the planning process take place at all three levels but it should also be one in which the mission and service departments under the guidance of SBU management participate in the development of the initial strategic plans. These plans then move up to the SBU level where SBU management develops them under the guidance of corporate management. The SBU plans then move up to the corporate management level, which then develops the overall strategic plans.

In contrast to that three-level planning process, many hospitals utilize a separate planning department headed by a planning director to do their strategic planning. However, strategic planning, to be successful, must be a multi-level joint activity involving full participation by all levels of management.

This chapter explores the (1) use of the mission and service department sectors in strategic planning, (2) the notions and needs of both rearward and forward vertical integration, (3) the benefits of horizontal integration, and (4) corporate reorganization.

DESCRIPTION OF A STRATEGIC BUSINESS UNIT (SBU)

The concept of the SBU was formalized with the advent of strategic planning by large corporations in the early 1970s. The notable leader in this area was the General Electric Corporation.

Although the term "SBU" only dates back to about 1970 the notion of an entity similar to the SBU has been around much longer. In earlier days SBUs

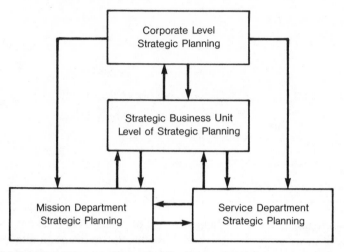

Figure 7-1 Schematic Diagram of Strategic Planning Levels in Health Care Organization

may have been called subsidiaries or major profit centers, although every subsidiary or profit center is not an SBU.

What is new in corporate strategic planning is the explicit segmentation of large corporations into SBUs, largely for strategic planning purposes, but also for management control. The concept of the SBU allows strategic planning to occur at the SBU level without the process necessarily affecting other SBUs. SBUs can also stand alone as viable and independent companies or divisions.

The definition of SBUs proposed by Rothschild lists a number of criteria that must be satisfied before an entity can be considered to be a SBU.[1] The first criterion is that an SBU must serve an external market; that is, it must have its own clientele. Second, it must have a clear group of external competitors with which it is vying for market share. Third, it must have reasonable control over its service delivery or manufacturing process, including the hiring and firing of employees. Fourth, the SBU performance must be measurable in terms of profits and losses. In other words, it must be a true revenue center.

Based on the above definition, the hospitals in a multihospital chain would clearly qualify as SBUs. Similarly, a local health care organization that owns two hospitals, a HMO, and a nursing home could segment the corporation into four SBUs.

DEFINITIONS OF A MISSION DEPARTMENT (MD) AND A
SERVICE DEPARTMENT (SD)

A mission department in a hospital or other health facility is a department or subunit that performs a unique patient service mission in the health facility. In performing the patient service mission, it may do so for external clients or for internal clients. As a mission department it has its own budget and its own billable clients.

Examples of mission departments in a hospital are the emergency room, the outpatient clinic, imaging center, laboratory, pharmacy, psychiatric clinic, physical therapy department, and occupational therapy department. Each of these departments could not only be located in hospitals but also in large ambulatory care centers, closed panel HMOs, and in nursing homes.

Most departments that serve the mission departments are considered service departments. Examples are housekeeping, billing, admissions, food service, and data processing. Service departments usually do not bill patients directly for services performed. If they do, then they may be viewed as mission departments. For instance, if a hospital bills its patients separately for hotel service and food service, then hotel service and food service could be considered mission departments.

The notion of a mission department is to a limited extent analogous to the previously described SBU. Therefore, to a limited extent the planning tools developed for SBU planning can also be used for mission department planning.

DEFINITION OF MISSION AND SERVICE DEPARTMENT
SECTORS IN CORPORATE PLANNING

The concept of mission and service department sectors in corporate strategic planning imposes a form of matrix organization onto the strategic planning activities of a multi-SBU corporation. The mission and service department sectors connect all special mission departments and service departments in all of the SBUs. This ensures that strategic planning assumptions and procedures will be similar in each mission or service department. However, each SBU can still do its own strategic planning.

A graphic example of how mission and service department sector planning operates is shown in Table 7-1. Note that each similar mission department or service department in each SBU is not only part of the SBU but also is part of the respective mission or service department sector. This arrangement is not only used for strategic planning but also for operations management, man-

Table 7-1 Matrix Organization for Strategic Planning,
Operations Management and Management Control

	SBU1	SBU2	SBU3	SBU4
MDS1	MD1	MD1	MD1	MD1
MDS2	MD2	MD2	MD2	MD2
SDS1	SD1	SD1	SD1	SD1
SDS2	SD2	SD2	SD2	SD2

Note: MD = Mission department
         SD = Service department
         SBU = Strategic business unit
         MDS = Mission department sector
         SDS = Service department sector

agement control, management training, centralized purchasing, and other activities that can benefit from coordination.

Table 7-2 shows how the mission departments and service departments in a typical multihospital chain appear in a matrix organization format. As can be seen, all pharmacy departments are part of the pharmacy sector, all physical therapy departments are part of the physical therapy sector, etc.

Mission department sectors and service department sectors provide considerable opportunities for economies of scale, sharing of expertise, and joint purchasing and training of personnel. These benefits of specialization reduce operating costs and require special approaches to strategic planning.

Table 7-2 Matrix Organization Using Sectors for a Typical Multihospital Corporation

	Olinda Hospital	Marks Hospital	Camino Hospital	Suburban Hospital
Pharmacy Sector	PD	PD	PD	PD
Physical Therapy Sector	PTD	PTD	PTD	PTD
Imaging Sector	ID	ID	ID	ID

Note: PD = Pharmacy department
         PTD = Physical therapy department
         ID = Imaging department

CORPORATE STRATEGIC PLANNING FOR HEALTH FACILITIES

Strategic planning at the corporate level should coordinate and guide the separate planning activities of the SBUs. Ideally, strategic planning is a collaborative activity whereby the (1) mission departments and service departments under the guidance of the mission department sectors and service department sectors, on the one hand, and the strategic SBUs, on the other hand, develop their respective strategic plans at the same time as (2) the SBUs develop their strategic plans for their respective units under the guidance of the corporate strategic planning department. Coordinating the activities of the mission department sector and service department sector is also a corporate-level responsibility. Exceptions to the above are those cases where new strategic units or mission departments are being developed, and most of the planning must emanate from the corporate strategic planning group.

Table 7-3 shows the participation of the various groups in the strategic planning process. Note that each SBU and the corporation as a whole has its own mission statement. All three levels—the corporation, SBU, and mission or service department—have their own set of objectives and strategies, including tactics and action plans.

The flow of information between the various groups in strategic planning is shown in Figure 7-2. Note that there are many lines of information between the corporate level and the SBU level, on the one hand, and between the SBU level and the mission or service department level, on the other hand. The important and initial lines of communication are those that flow upward from the mission and service departments to the SBUs and from the SBUs to the corporate level.

Table 7-3 Relationship of Corporate Strategic Planning to SBU and Mission or Service Department Strategic Planning

	Mission	Goals	Objectives	Strategy	
				Tactics	Action Plans
Corporation	x	x	x	x	x
Strategic Business Unit	x	x	x	x	x
Mission Department		x	x	x	x
Service Department		x	x	x	x

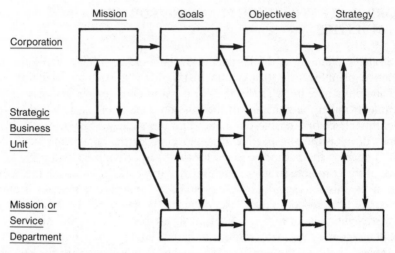

Figure 7-2 Information Flows among the Corporation, the SBUs, and the Mission or Service Departments

GENERIC STRATEGIES FOR CORPORATE PLANNING

Porter has proposed three "generic" strategies for corporations: cost leadership, differentiation, and focus.[2] These three strategies also have important implications for health care corporations.

Multihealth care facility organizations, such as hospital chains, integrated health networks, nursing home chains, and multi-unit HMOs, may particularly want to consider the cost leadership strategy. By using the mission department sector approach discussed in the previous section, these corporations are able to be more cost-effective through specialization, economies of scale, sharing of expertise, and joint training and purchasing activities. In this age of increasing competition in the health care sector the ability to compete on a cost-price basis is becoming more critical for retaining or improving market share and profitability.

The differentiation strategy is another important consideration not only for the large multifacility health care organizations but also for the larger local integrated health facilities. The most logical way to utilize the differentiation strategy is through the use of a brand name. Organizations in the health insurance field that have used this extensively are Blue Cross and Blue Shield. More recently, the Humana health care corporation is using "Humana" as its brand name for the various health care services it markets. This would not be possible if it had not first established a national presence through its artificial heart program in Louisville. The Mayo Clinic is another organization that capitalizes on name recognition.

The focus strategy has been and still is extensively used by special market niches in the health care market, such as psychiatric hospitals and alcohol and drug rehabilitation centers. Another focus area is the convenient ambulatory care center such as "urgent care" or freestanding "emergency" centers.

VERTICAL INTEGRATION

Rearward Vertical Integration

Increasingly, many hospitals are actively involved in or are planning to engage in rearward vertical integration. The driving force for rearward vertical integration is the increasing competition among hospitals to retain or expand market share.

Rearward vertical integration is defined as the creation or acquisition of new SBUs that further develop distribution channels and strengthen the flow of patient referrals into the hospital. The typical example of rearward vertical integration is the development or acquisition of ambulatory care centers and/ or HMOs. Through these rearward vertical integration efforts hospitals are able to increase their share of hospital admissions and ancillary services, thus achieving increased revenues.

Rearward vertical integration can be used both to strengthen market share in current service areas and develop new service areas. It is often a strategy that follows a particular product line and/or brand name recognition campaign. For example, the hospital choosing to promote its women's services program may set up a freestanding ambulatory center in an area of strategic importance. That center would offer mammography, osteoporosis screening, PMS counseling, and other specific services that women could gain access to directly or on referral from a private physician.

Competition is a key concern of any rearward vertical integration process because the hospital is entering into fields of care that are not necessarily in its original domain. This expansion could arouse the opposition of the medical staff and competing hospitals. The reaction of the medical staff must be of greatest concern, as no hospital can risk the total alienation of its greatest referral source! Therefore, inclusion of medical staff in the planning process is a tactic that *every* hospital should follow. That inclusion, however, is not generally sufficient. Great pains should be taken to present potentially sensitive projects in a manner that shows their benefits for physicians. Often, the hospital may offer a business joint venture to physicians that would allow them to profit from the success of the new program. Physicians should be so involved in the planning process that they are in the position of "selling" the new service to other physicians; management and/or board members are often perceived as a threat to the economic interests of physicians.

Competition with other area hospitals is a different issue that requires different approaches. In this case it becomes a matter of the regional health plan developed by the local planning agency and often comes down to the survival of one of the institutions. Although competition among hospitals is usually an expensive proposition for communities (duplication of capital investment and services, etc.) the regulatory environment of the 1980s appears to be moving toward that approach for developing the natural health care system. The major point is to discuss openly the corporate philosophy of competition and/or cooperation with neighboring hospitals so as to avoid espousing one strategy while pursuing another.

A rearward vertical integration strategy has both opportunities and pitfalls. Detailed planning and feasibility analysis must be performed before such a strategy is undertaken.

Forward Vertical Integration

The strategy of forward vertical integration is also being adopted by many hospitals in order to retain a larger portion of the health care dollar being expended. Forward vertical integration is accomplished through the development or acquisition of nursing homes and home health care organizations, both of which provide posthospital care. Under the prospective payment system of diagnostic-related groupings, a hospital with a home health care unit can simultaneously provide continuity of care and retain a larger share of the health care dollar. Many systems are even moving into housing and long-term home health care programs.

Ownership of nursing homes is another way to accomplish forward vertical integration. Patients entering nursing homes usually do so after a stay in an acute health care facility. Hence, transferring a patient from the hospital to its own nursing home also enables the hospital to provide continuity of care and also retain a larger portion of the health care dollar.

Forward vertical integration, as opposed to rearward vertical integration, does not usually alienate physicians. As a result it is a safer strategy to pursue. It is the strategy of choice for the major national health care provider corporations. However, the more critical strategy for individual hospitals—the one that captures market share—is rearward vertical integration. Figure 7-3 shows both forms of vertical integration.

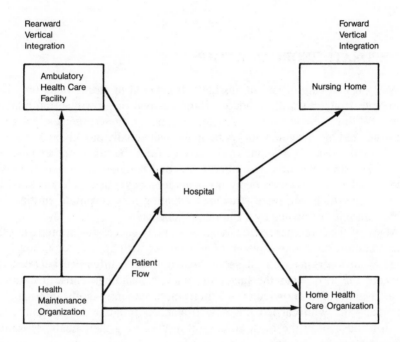

Figure 7-3 Rearward and Forward Vertical Integration

HORIZONTAL INTEGRATION

Horizontal integration is an expansion process that is focused on activities in which the corporation is currently engaged. A multinursing home chain is probably the most common example of a horizontally integrated system. Individual hospitals planning to or engaged in acquiring other hospitals or merging with other hospitals are engaging in horizontal integration.

The major benefit of horizontal integration is the potential of economies of scale of support operations, such as purchasing, data processing, and billing. Specialization and standardization are other benefits of horizontal integration. It can both lower costs and also lead to higher quality service. By utilizing a brand name for the type of health care being delivered, horizontal integration also allows the development of a differentiation strategy.

The success of multihospital chains in lowering costs in comparison with individual stand-alone hospitals clearly indicates that the future trend is in the direction of more horizontal integration for hospitals, nursing homes, and HMOs.

CORPORATE REORGANIZATION

Many health care organizations have discovered in recent years that their corporate structures are not adequate for survival or growth in the marketplace. With the environment changing so quickly, these organizations must be structured in a way that allows them to react equally quickly and that also insulates the risks of any one business unit from that of the other business units. The strategies of vertical and horizontal integration opened new avenues for change, of which many hospitals took advantage. They reacted by reorganizing their corporate structures, creating new corporate entities that were controlled or owned by a central power center.

Many of these reorganizations were extremely successful in preparing the corporation for a competitive environment. As with any strategy, however, there were losers as well. It seems that the main difference between the winners and losers was the factor of strategic planning. Those institutions with a thorough knowledge of their environments—both internal and external—and who carried out a well-planned program of reorganization seem to have been the most successful at achieving their goals. Hospitals reorganizing only because their competition was doing so—how often we saw this phenomenon!—with no clear direction or commitment, got lost in the process and often failed. Many reorganizations were subsequently reorganized to correct initial mistakes. Other very successful hospitals discovered that reorganization would not be helpful to achieving their goals and in fact have been very successful without it. Therefore, one must look very carefully at the strategy of corporate reorganization as a means of implementing programs that meet the perceived threat of new competition in the industry or marketplace.

Figure 7-4 shows a typical corporate reorganization for not-for-profit hospitals in the United States as part of their pursuit of a broader base of economic support. In this basic model of reorganization, a parent corporation is created with a mission that is broader based than that of a hospital. The parent creates a foundation subsidiary for the sole purpose of raising funds in support of the hospital. A for-profit business (or businesses) is wholly owned by the parent corporation and is developed in a manner that enables quick entry into related fields of endeavor, such as home health care, ambulatory surgery, and skilled nursing. The advantage of this model is that the parent's mission can be broadened to include almost anything that will help ultimately support the hospital, thus preserving intact the hospital's original mission.

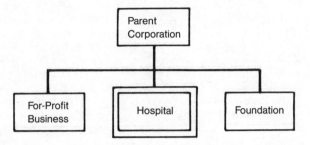

Figure 7-4 Typical Reorganization for a Not-for-Profit Hospital

The biggest disadvantage is the eventual loss of some control by the not-for-profit hospital and the loss by that hospital of the direct income from the new ventures. This model reflects a long-term focus in pursuit of capital development where the parent corporation is relegated to that of conduit of funds and organizer.

A second popular model for reorganization is a strong hospital model, wherein the hospital maintains its status as the parent corporation while developing its supporting subsidiaries as shown in Figure 7-5. As a simpler model, this particular approach sacrifices flexibility for control. A third model, shown in Figure 7-6, is sometimes called the foundation model; in it a foundation is established as the parent corporation with the purpose of creating enterprises that develop a capital base for the hospital.

Even the simplest structural change can have a major impact on the success of a hospital's ventures. The strategic planning process for entering into new avenues must therefore take a long-range view and consider far more than the first one or two ventures when determining the appropriate structure for the hospital.

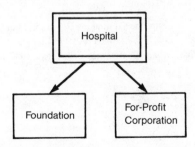

Figure 7-5 Reorganization with Strong Hospital Model

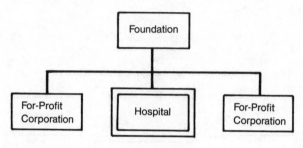

Figure 7-6 Foundation Model of Hospital Reorganization

SUMMARY

The matrix organizational format has been presented as a model for strategic planning for multi-SBU health care corporations. The columns in the matrix model represent the various SBUs of the corporation, and the rows represent the mission and service department sectors of the corporation. The matrix model is useful for both strategic planning and for management control.

The structural change in hospital reimbursement from cost-based to prospective payment is forcing hospitals to review their strategies and structure. Both rearward and forward vertical integration are required to ensure that the hospital of the future can remain competitive and retain its market share.

The three levels of planning are corporate level strategic planning, SBU strategic planning, and mission or service department strategic planning. All management levels should participate in the planning process. Full participation by management facilitates implementation of the strategic plan.

The organization must be structured in a manner that reacts to, rather than drives, corporate strategies.

NOTES

1. W.E. Rothschild, "How to Insure the Continuous Growth in Strategic Planning," *The Journal of Business Strategy,* 1, no. 1 (Summer 1980):11–18.

2. M. E. Porter, *Competitive Strategy* (New York: Free Press, 1980,), Chapters 3–5.

Financial and Operating Ratio Analysis

8

This chapter reviews how financial and operating ratios can be used to evaluate the financial and operating status of health care institutions. Four types of ratios—liquidity, profitability, leverage, and operating ratios—are presented (Exhibit 8-1).

Liquidity ratios include the current ratio, the quick ratio, and the cash ratio. Profitability ratios include return on assets, return on equity, and return on revenues. Leverage ratios include the debt-equity ratio, the long-term debt-equity ratio, and the long-term debt-total assets ratio. Operating ratios include the inventory turnover ratio, the accounts receivable turnover ratio, and the assets turn over ratio.

The above ratios are then applied to four hospitals in order to obtain a cross-sectional analysis and to one large multihospital system to obtain a time-series comparison. Finally, the chapter discusses an approach to determining the financial viability of a hospital.

DEFINITION OF THE FINANCIAL AND OPERATING RATIOS

Liquidity Ratios

The most important liquidity ratio is the current ratio. It is defined as:

$$\text{Current Ratio} = \frac{\text{Current Assets}}{\text{Current Liabilities}}$$

The current ratio measures the ratio of assets that can be converted into cash quickly—within 1 year or less—to the debts that have to be paid within 1 year. Because the ratio is measured at a point in time—say, at the end of a

Exhibit 8-1 Summary of Financial Operating Ratios

Liquidity Ratios
  Current ratio
  Quick ratio
  Cash ratio
Leverage Ratios
  Debt-equity ratio
  Long-term debt-equity ratio
  Long-term debt-total assets ratio
Profitability Ratios
  Return on assets
  Return on equity
  Return on revenues
Operating Ratios
  Inventory turnover ratio
  Accounts receivable turnover ratio
  Assets turnover ratio

---

fiscal period—it only provides a snapshot of the organization's financial condition. However, the snapshot is fairly accurate. The ratio should be higher than 1.0 and preferably about 2.0. The minimum ratio varies from industry to industry, but is generally between 1.0 and 2.0.

The quick ratio has a different numerator than the current ratio. The numerator of the quick ratio consists of current assets less inventory. Because inventory in a health care situation is *usually* relatively low, the two ratios are usually quite similar. The quick ratio is defined as:

$$\text{Quick Ratio} = \frac{\text{Current Assets} - \text{Inventory}}{\text{Current Liabilities}}$$

In the cash ratio, cash or marketable securities are in the numerator, rather than current assets. The cash ratio measures what percent of liabilities that are due within 1 year can be paid immediately. It is to some extent a measure of how conservative management is in its short-term assets management. The cash ratio is defined as:

$$\text{Cash Ratio} = \frac{\text{Cash} + \text{Marketable Securities}}{\text{Current Liabilities}}$$

Profitability Ratios

The first profitability ratio, the return on assets ratio, is defined as:

$$\text{Return on Assets Ratio} = \frac{\text{Net Income after Tax}}{\text{Total Assets}}$$

The return on assets ratio measures the rate of return that the hospital earns on all of its assets. It is a good ratio for comparison purposes. However, if the hospital has incurred heavy debt, this ratio will be relatively low because the net income is based on the amount available after interest is paid.

The second profitability ratio is the return on equity ratio. It is defined as:

$$\text{Return on Equity Ratio} = \frac{\text{Net Income after Tax}}{\text{Total Equity}}$$

The return on equity ratio measures the profitability of the hospital more fairly than the return on assets ratio because it is based on the return that is earned by investors on their investment or, in the case of a nonprofit hospital, what the institution has earned on its investment in the hospital.

The third profitability ratio, the return on revenue ratio, is defined as:

$$\text{Return on Revenue Ratio} = \frac{\text{Net Income after Tax}}{\text{Total Revenue}}$$

The return on revenue ratio provides a measure of the net margin earned on revenues. In an investor-owned hospital the net margin has to be high enough to attract investors in the hospital corporation. The net margin of a nonprofit hospital must be sufficient to allow for capital formation, ensuring continued growth and modernization of the hospital or expansion into new services.

Leverage Ratios

The three leverage ratios measure the ratios of debt to assets and equity. The first leverage ratio is the most commonly used one. It is the debt-equity ratio and is defined as:

$$\text{Debt-Equity Ratio} = \frac{\text{Total Liabilities}}{\text{Total Equity}}$$

The second leverage ratio is the long-term debt to equity ratio. It is defined as:

$$\text{Long-Term Debt-Equity Ratio} = \frac{\text{Long-Term Debt}}{\text{Total Equity}}$$

Both the debt-equity and long-term debt-equity ratios measure the stability of the hospital's longer-term financial status. High ratios indicate that the probability of financial difficulty and possibly bankruptcy is increased because debt will have to be repaid at some future time. Low ratios are an indicator of conservative long-term financial management.

The third leverage ratio, which is the long-term debts to assets ratio, is defined as:

$$\text{Long-Term Debt-Assets Ratio} = \frac{\text{Long-Term Debt}}{\text{Total Assets}}$$

The long-term debt-assets ratio measures the proportion of the assets that are financed by long-term debt. Again, the lower the figure, the better.

Operating Ratios

The three operating ratios measure how well the assets are utilized. The first operating ratio, the inventory turnover ratio, is defined as:

$$\text{Inventory Turnover Ratio} = \frac{\text{Total Revenues}}{\text{Inventory}}$$

The inventory turnover ratio indicates the level of inventory that is kept available in the hospital. The higher this ratio, the more efficient the hospital inventory management because unneeded inventory kept on hand incurs unnecessary capital and insurance charges and may be subject to wastage and pilferage.

The second operating ratio is the accounts receivable turnover ratio. It is defined as:

$$\text{Accounts Receivable Turnover Ratio} = \frac{\text{Total Revenues}}{\text{Accounts Receivable}}$$

The accounts receivable ratio indicates how quickly patients and third parties pay their bills. The ideal ratio is 12 because it indicates that all bills on average are paid monthly. This ideal is, however, seldom attained by even the most effective hospital.

The third operating ratio, the assets turnover ratio, is defined as:

$$\text{Assets Turnover Ratio} = \frac{\text{Total Revenues}}{\text{Total Assets}}$$

The assets turnover ratio measures the proportion of revenues to total assets. Generally, annual revenues should at least equal total assets. Unfortunately, that ideal is not always attainable.

TIME-SERIES ANALYSIS OF FINANCIAL AND OPERATING RATIOS

To see how these ratios can be used to evaluate the performance of a hospital or health-related corporation, a time-series analysis is made of Humana Inc., a publicly held multi-institutional health service corporation that operates hospitals, HMOs, health insurance firms, and other health-related facilities.

From annual reports was constructed a 7-year overview of the financial and operating performance of Humana. Table 8-1 shows the 12 financial and operating ratios from the years 1979 to 1985. Reviewing the financial and

Table 8-1 Time-Series Analysis of Financial and Operating Ratios of Humana Inc., 1979–1985

	1979	1980	1981	1982	1983	1984	1985
Liquidity Ratios							
Current ratio	1.49	1.39	1.41	1.56	1.71	1.72	1.48
Quick ratio	1.35	1.25	1.31	1.43	1.58	1.59	1.34
Cash ratio	0.61	0.57	0.72	0.77	0.82	0.74	0.23
Profitability Ratios							
Return on assets	0.038	0.054	0.068	0.073	0.072	0.075	0.079
Return on equity	0.174	0.229	0.258	0.330	0.264	0.260	0.239
Return on revenue	0.036	0.046	0.055	0.066	0.070	0.074	0.075
Leverage Ratios							
Debt-equity	4.06	3.70	3.16	2.92	2.31	2.47	2.01
Long-term debt—equity	2.98	2.56	2.03	2.30	1.86	1.99	1.61
Long-term debt—assets	0.59	0.54	0.49	0.59	0.56	0.57	0.53
Operating Ratios							
Inventory turnover	49.3	48.9	56.8	56.0	55.4	57.6	56.5
Accts. rec. turnover	9.7	10.8	11.4	11.5	11.5	10.1	7.9
Assets turnover	0.94	1.05	1.13	1.10	1.04	1.01	1.06

operating ratios over the 7 years allows one to evaluate how well an organization has performed and to project reasonable estimates of future performance for strategic planning purposes.

Note that the current ratio has ranged from a low of 1.39 to a high of 1.72. The 1985 current ratio of 1.48 therefore provides no reason for concern. The quick ratio has ranged from 1.25 to 1.59. The 1985 quick ratio of 1.34 is therefore also acceptable. The only liquidity ratio of some concern is the cash ratio, which ranged from 0.23 in 1985 to 0.82. One would want to investigate why it is so low in 1985.

The profitability ratios can be similarly reviewed. The return on assets ratio has increased on an almost consistent basis from a low in 1979 of 0.038 to its current high of 0.079 in 1985. The return on equity ratio has ranged from 0.174 to 0.330. Its 1985 figure is 0.239, still well within the range. However, since 1982 the return on assets ratio has been increasing while the return on equity has decreased from 0.330 in 1982 to 0.239 in 1985. This decrease has probably been caused by management's decision to decrease its debt-equity ratio (see below). The return on revenue ratio has steadily increased from a low of 0.036 in 1979 to a high of 0.075 in 1985. A steady increase over a 7-year period usually indicates that the organization is well managed.

The leverage ratios indicate that management has been decreasing its debt-equity ratios during the 7-year period. The debt-equity ratio declined from 4.06 in 1979 to a low of 2.01 in 1985. Similarly, the long-term debt-equity ratio also declined from 2.98 in 1979 to a low of 1.61 in 1985. The long-term debt-assets ratio has been more stable over the 7-year period, during which time it has ranged from 0.49 to 0.59. In 1985 the long-term debt-equity ratio was 0.53, a figure well within this rather narrow range.

The operating ratios in general were quite stable. The inventory turnover ratio ranged from 48.9 to 57.6. The 1985 ratio of 56.6 is well within the range, although near the higher end, which is desirable. The accounts receivable turnover ratio ranged from 7.9 to 11.5. The lowest and least desirable figure was attained in 1985. Although the low figure of 7.9 is no cause for serious concern, it certainly should be investigated. The assets turnover ratio ranged from 0.94 to 1.13. The 1985 assets turnover ratio of 1.06 is well within the range and appears normal for the mix of health-related businesses in which Humana Inc. is engaged.

CROSS-SECTIONAL ANALYSIS OF FINANCIAL AND OPERATING RATIOS

A cross-sectional analysis of financial and operating ratios is now performed for four community hospitals ranging in size from 160 to 240 beds. A summary of the twelve ratios for the four hospitals is shown in Table 8-2. Cross-sectional analysis allows comparison between several hospitals and facilitates the identification of exceptions to the norm that may be in a desirable or undesirable direction.

Note that all current ratios are quite acceptable. The lowest is 1.94 and the highest is 2.78. Similarly the quick ratios are also quite acceptable as they fall in a range from 1.78 to 2.61. However, the cash ratio of Bayview Community hospital is quite low at 0.11. Management clearly would want to investigate how this ratio can be improved.

Improving the current, quick, and cash ratios is of immediate concern to hospital management whenever these ratios fall below acceptable levels. Actions to improve these ratios focus on the cash account. An increase in the cash account through an inflow of cash from outside the corporation that would not affect the other current accounts will improve all ratios. Achieving such an increase may require, however, a long-term loan, a cash bequest, or a sale of equity in the for-profit corporation.

A temporary "fix" that improves the cash ratio can be accomplished by actively changing the composition of the current accounts. For instance, delaying the time by which you pay your bills will improve the cash account somewhat, but will probably hurt your credit rating. Similarly, urging your customers to pay their bills earlier than normal will improve your cash ratio,

Table 8-2 Cross-Sectional Analysis of Financial and Operating Ratios for Four Community Hospitals in 1985

	Lansford Community Hospital	Metropolitan General Hospital	Suburban General Hospital	Bayview Community Hospital
Liquidity Ratios				
Current ratio	2.20	2.16	2.78	1.94
Quick ratio	1.78	2.01	2.61	1.80
Cash ratio	0.35	0.37	0.76	0.11
Profitability Ratios				
Return on assets	0.023	0.021	0.084	0.043
Return on equity	0.037	0.060	0.128	0.125
Return on revenue	0.023	0.033	0.081	0.065
Leverage Ratios				
Debt-equity	0.56	1.91	0.51	1.89
Long-term debt—equity	0.40	1.74	0.33	1.63
Long-term debt—assets	0.26	0.60	0.22	0.56
Operating Ratios				
Inventory turnover	24.3	71.3	50.6	51.7
Accts. rec. turnover	8.7	6.9	4.7	4.4
Assets turnover	1.02	0.62	1.04	0.69

but may also result in poor customer relations. One of the more effective methods that hospitals have used to improve the quick and cash ratio is by reducing inventory. Inventory reduction indirectly makes more cash available and thus improves the ratios.

The profitability ratios indicate that all hospitals have at least a satisfactory profitability level as measured by all three ratios. However, the profitability of Suburban General Hospital is higher than the others, and Bayview Community is definitely in a better position than the two lower profitability hospitals.

The leverage ratios also show substantial variance. Two hospitals, Lansford Community and Suburban General Hospitals, show more conservative long-term financial policies in comparison with the more risky long-term financial policies of Metropolitan General and Bayview Community Hospitals.

Improving profitability and leverage ratios are issues addressed by this entire book. If the profitability and leverage ratios are unsatisfactory, then a major priority in strategic development should be to improve these ratios. Slight improvements in profitability can frequently be achieved by short-term actions aimed at increasing efficiency and achieving cost reductions. Major improvements in profitability, however, frequently require changes in case mix, changes in physician affiliations, acquisition of new and high technology equipment, changes or expansion of physical facilities, or the like. These major changes nearly always require capital investments and can only be accomplished over a multiyear period.

Related to an institution's profitability are of course the leverage ratios. If leverage is already too high, then it can become a major barrier to many of the required changes, such as acquisition of new technology equipment or expansion of facilities. For-profit corporations frequently are at some advantage because they may be able to raise at least some of the needed capital through the sale of part of the equity in the corporation.

The greatest divergence in any category of ratios is seen in the operating ratios. A rather low inventory turnover ratio is shown for Lansford Community Hospital, and it probably should be investigated. The accounts receivable turnover ratio is particularly low for Suburban General and Bayview Community Hospitals. The ratios are 4.7 and 4.4, which means that bills on average are paid at 78 and 83 days, respectively. Such delays in bill payments could considerably strain a hospital's finances and could also possibly indicate that an above-average proportion of accounts receivable is bad debt. The asset turnover ratio is quite acceptable for two hospitals, but is too low for Metropolitan General at 0.62 and for Bayview Community Hospital at 0.69. The rather inefficient utilization of the two hospitals' assets should be investigated.

FINANCIAL VIABILITY OF A HOSPITAL

This discussion grew out of the participation by one of the authors on a community task force that had as its mandate the evaluation of the financial soundness of 36 acute care hospitals. The resource person assigned to the task force had developed 29 financial ratios for each of the 36 hospitals, and it was the task force's responsibility to evaluate these financial ratios and make recommendations about those ratios that were relevant.

The result was a model, developed by the author, to summarize much of the financial information contained in the respective organizations' financial statements into a single index. This single index was named a financial viability index.[1] It is based on three financial ratios:

1. Capital structure ratio

$$\text{Assets financed by liabilities (AFL)} = \frac{\text{Long-Term Debt}}{\text{Total Assets}}$$

2. Liquidity ratio:

$$\text{Critical ratio (CR)} = \frac{\text{Current Assets}}{\text{Current Liabilities}}$$

3. Profitability ratio:

$$\text{Operating expense to Operating revenue ratio (OER)} = \frac{\text{Total Operating Expenses}}{\text{Total Operating Revenue}}$$

The value of a single financial viability index has been recognized for a long time. A single index, provided of course that it is valid, makes it much easier to compare the financial condition of an organization with the financial status of other organizations.

In the hospital field, Caruana and Kudder[2] and the Alpha Center for Health Planning[3] proposed use of a single index to measure the financial viability of a hospital. This index called α, is derived according to the formula

$$\alpha = \frac{4(\text{AFL})(\text{OER})^4}{\text{CR}}$$

where AFL, OER, and CR are as defined before. The α financial viability index measures (1) short-term financial status position with the current ratio (CR), (2) the long-term debt position with the ratio of assets divided by liabilities (AFL), and (3) the profitability measure with the ratio of operating expenses divided by operating revenue (OER).

However, because three ratios must be multiplied to calculate the index, incorrect values tend to be generated if any one of the three ratios is an extremely low or extremely high figure. Because extreme values are quite common, especially for the first two ratios, the frequency of incorrect values for the α index is quite common.

The proposed alternative to the α index uses a discrete function of the same three financial ratios in an additive combination. Using a discrete function eliminates the extremely low or high values of the individual ratios, and making the discrete functions additive ensures that they are equally weighted.

The functional form for the three financial ratios—CR, AFL, and OER—is shown in Table 8-3. Note that in each case the functional value of each ratio is indexed on an integer scale from 0 to 5. The mapping of the ratios onto the integral values was performed by a group of eight hospital financial experts. Within the scale that is from 1 to 4 the integral values are also linearly related to the values of the respective ratio. Hence, a considerable amount of validity can be claimed for the proposed financial viability index.

For each hospital the three scaled values were added to make a total score or index. This index was named the β index to differentiate it from the α index. Theoretically, the β index can range from 0-15.

Application of Viability Index

The two financial viability indexes—the α and β indexes, were used to analyze the financial data of 36 hospitals in a large metropolitan area. For each of the 36 hospitals, financial ratios for CR, AFL, and OER were collected as shown on Table 8-4. Each of the ratios was converted onto the 0-5 viability measurement scale, and the scaled values were summed to provide

Table 8-3 Functions of CR, AFL, and OER

CR	f(CR)	AFL	f(AFL)	OER	f(OER)
<1.0	0	>.600	0	>1.04	0
>1.0–<1.3	1	>.500–<.600	1	>1.03–<1.04	1
>1.3–<1.6	2	>.400–<.500	2	>1.02–<1.03	2
>1.6–<1.9	3	>.300–<.400	3	>1.01–<1.02	3
>1.9–<2.2	4	>.200–<.300	3	>1.00–<1.01	4
>2.2	5	<.200	5	<1.00	5

Note: CR = critical ratio
AFL = assets financed by liabilities
OER = ratio of operating expenses to operating revenues

Table 8-4 Actual and Functional Values of Three Financial Ratios

Hospital	CR	f(CR)	AFL	f(AFL)	OER	f(OER)	β Index	α Index
A	2.471	5	.408	2	1.013	3	10	.695
B	1.177	1	.521	1	1.019	3	5	1.909
C	1.875	3	.312	3	1.007	4	10	.684
D	2.104	4	.211	4	1.055	0	8	.497
E	1.509	2	.479	2	1.039	1	5	1.480
F	2.655	5	.210	4	1.002	4	13	.319
G	1.245	1	.559	1	1.049	0	2	2.175
H	2.459	5	.256	4	1.009	4	13	.432
I	1.563	2	.355	3	1.029	2	7	1.019
J	3.176	5	.387	3	1.001	4	12	.489
K	13.828	5	.377	3	1.320	5	13	.331
L	1.052	1	.542	1	1.004	4	6	2.094
M	.968	0	.410	2	1.063	0	2	1.163
N	1.625	3	.764	0	1.054	0	3	3.038
O	9.524	5	.118	5	1.015	3	13	.053
P	2.813	5	.087	5	.968	5	15	.109
Q	.875	0	.945	0	1.206	2	2	9.138
R	1.364	2	.884	0	1.019	3	5	2.795
S	1.976	4	.146	5	.987	5	14	.280
T	2.002	4	.453	2	1.024	2	8	.995
U	1.777	3	.389	3	1.042	0	6	1.032
V	1.811	3	.666	0	1.006	4	7	1.507
W	1.962	4	.404	2	.990	5	11	.791
X	1.916	4	.506	1	1.010	3	8	1.099
Y	1.210	1	.354	3	1.067	0	4	1.517
Z	3.055	5	.166	5	1.022	2	12	.237
AA	1.485	2	.663	0	1.015	3	5	1.895
BB	2.543	5	.160	5	1.006	4	14	.258
CC	1.813	3	.258	4	1.009	4	11	.590
DD	1.262	1	.274	4	1.114	3	8	1.211
EE	3.481	5	.209	4	1.006	4	14	.246
FF	1.963	4	.592	1	1.006	4	9	1.236
GG	4.234	5	.066	5	1.015	3	13	.066
HH	2.204	5	.543	1	1.030	1	7	1.109
II	2.484	5	.221	4	1.118	0	9	.500
JJ	1.473	2	.402	2	1.019	3	7	1.177

the β index. A high β index value indicates a very strong financial position. A very low β index value indicates a poor financial position for the respective hospital.

In order to make the β index more meaningful, the index was categorized, and each category was labeled as shown in Table 8-5. The labels used were subjectively determined and generated considerable consternation, especially for those hospitals that fell in the grave and poor financial condition categories. The labeling can, of course, be modified to appear more generous. This

Table 8-5 Categorization of Alternative Financial Viability Indexes

Alternative Financial Index (β)	Financial Condition
0	
1	Grave
2	
3	
4	
5	Poor
6	
7	
8	Weak
9	
10	
11	Reasonable
12	
13	
14	Good
15	

was not done in this particular case because the intent of the study was to draw attention to the financially precarious position of some of the hospitals.

One would expect a high negative correlation between the α and β indexes. To test this hypothesis a correlation test was run on the two indexes. As expected, the correlation was quite high. The R^2 was .424, and the determination index was $-.651$.

SUMMARY

With the stress on health care cost containment and the consistently highly scrutinized Medicare and Medicaid hospital claims, it is not surprising that many hospitals find themselves in precarious financial straits. The financial condition of a hospital is not always fully understood by hospital governance boards, and a uniform way of assessing the financial health of a hospital would be a helpful addition to the governance function of many hospitals.

The financial indexes discussed and proposed in this chapter provide the means by which hospital management and hospital board members can compare the financial condition of their hospital with the financial condition of other hospitals in its respective geographic region.

The proposed financial viability index is a suggested way to describe the financial condition of any hospital. Although one may quarrel with such terms as "grave" and "poor," any hospital that finds itself in this category should act quickly to get its financial house in order.

NOTES

1. C. Carl Pegels, "A Model for Evaluating Financial Viability of a Hospital," *Third International Conference on System Science in Health Care*, W. van Eimeren, R. Engelbrecht, C. D. Hagle (Eds.), Berlin, Heidelberg: Springer Verlag, 1984, 701–704.

2. R.A. Caruana, and G. Kudder, "Seeing through the Figures with Ratios," *Hospital Financial Management, June 1978, 6.*

3. Alpha Center for Health Planning, *The Analysis of Hospital Financial Viability,* April 1979, 16–29.

Chapter 9

Corporate Cultures and Business Strategy

HIGHLIGHTS

- Introduction
- Definition and Background
- Diagnosis—How To Analyze Cultures
- Leadership and the Organizational Culture
- Changing the Organizational Culture
- Future Cultures
- Studies
- Application Strategies
- Summary

9

INTRODUCTION

The major buzz words in health care today are reorganize, reconceptualize, and restructure. Changes in corporate organization are essential if health facilities are to maintain their fiscal strength and market position in an era of cost containment. Many health management companies (SamCor and Intermountain) have responded by making changes in their organizational structures. John Naisbitt's book *Megatrends* details 10 irreversible social trends.[1] Each trend suggests changes in the delivery of health services. Naisbitt asks managers to completely reconceptualize the nature of their businesses.

Robert Reich argues that America's strength—the way the nation organizes itself for production—threatens its decline.[2] He charges that America has failed to adapt to the worldwide reorganization of production. America's basic steel, automobile, and textile reliance on high volume standardized production must give way to more flexible systems of production. Under such systems, there are major changes in organizational structure, management-labor relations, and performance appraisal. In essence, he calls for a fundamental restructuring of American industry.

Corporate reorganization is a fundamental and far-reaching change in any firm. Not a simple midcourse correction, this activity requires that people throughout an organization change previous behavior patterns. New power relationships are formed, and there are the inevitable "winners and losers."

Corporate cultures have been depicted as an enormously potent means of bringing people together, while also serving as equally significant obstacles

Note: Reprinted from "Corporate Cultures and Business Strategy: A Health Management Company Perspective" by M. O. Bice, *Hospital & Health Services Administration*, Vol. 29, No. 4, pp. 64–78, with permission of the Foundation of the American College of Healthcare Executives, July/August © 1984.

to change. Culture is capable of blunting or significantly altering the intended impact of changes in an organization. I concluded that I could not reorganize the nature of my business without first understanding and then altering the existing corporate culture.

DEFINITION AND BACKGROUND

A corporate philosophy, according to Ouchi, includes the organization's objectives, its operating procedures, and its social and economic environmental constraints.[3] This philosophy leads to the development of smaller practices and modes of conduct that become a corporate culture. Maccoby stresses defining a work group's mission and values as a first step in a manager's learning process.[4] In any change process, one needs bedrock to stand upon. The first step is to define what should *not* change. Everything else is open to examination. He contends that people will experiment if they are assured that their basic values will be protected.

Culture is a pattern of beliefs and expectations shared by the organization's members.[5] These beliefs and expectations produce norms that shape the behavior of both individuals and groups within an organization. Culture is usually long-term, strategic, and difficult to change. It is rooted in beliefs and values. Cultures are a "more or less enduring constellation of forces within the group or organization that causes its members to respond in specific ways to a defined entity."[6] This definition suggests that cultures have a sustaining quality, but are not permanently fixed. An organizational culture[7] also represents the shared sense of the "way we do things around here," a critical factor in guiding day-to-day behavior and shaping a future course of action.

The notion of corporate culture is not new. Writing about the functions of the executive in 1938, Chester Barnard indicated that one of an executive's key functions was to manage and shape his company's values.[8] In 1957, Philip Selznick argued that the institutional leader is an expert in the promotion and protection of values.[9] More recently, writers such as Schwartz and Davis, Deal, Kennedy, Spiegel, and Peters have focused on corporate culture, management activities, and business strategies, leading to three basic conclusions:

- All businesses have cultures.
- Businesses with strong, environmentally relevant cultures perform better than others.
- Corporate cultures can be shaped, managed, and changed.

There are five cultural elements in both primitive and modern organizations[10]:

- Values and beliefs about success in the environment
- Heroes who epitomize those values and beliefs
- Rituals that prescribe how all critical activities are to be carried out
- Stories and storytellers to keep the mythology of the culture alive

The values and beliefs of a strong culture company are internalized and widely shared throughout the organization. These values are held with conviction by the organization's members and have long-term staying power. The company's heroes are people throughout the organization who, by their actions and impact on others, epitomize the firm's values and beliefs. Rituals reinforce values. There is a direct linkage between a daily or weekly activity and a key company value. These rituals are performed frequently, and participants understand and support the activity. Major and minor ceremonies help celebrate heroes and corporate achievements. The CEO is actively involved in these ceremonies, and significant corporate resources are invested. And finally, a rich organizational mythology is a sure sign of a culture that is alive and healthy.

Finding strong cultures in the business world is difficult enough. Hospitals with excellent cultures are even rarer.[11] A hospital has a variety of subcultures—the governing body, physicians, nursing, and departmental subcultures. So, a hospital is a hodgepodge of individual subcultures—some weak, some internally focused, and some externally focused—all of which must be knit together if the institution is to carry out its mission. Welding these subcultures together, by finding themes that channel efforts in a common direction, is a challenge that few hospitals can successfully meet. Hospital chains that grow by acquisition take on new entities that have developed unique cultures and philosophies, exacerbating the problem even more. In most instances, hospital cultures are weak, fragmented, and in need of attention.

DIAGNOSIS—HOW TO ANALYZE CULTURES

Authors have proposed different methods for analyzing corporate culture. Schwartz and Davis offer a cultural risk assessment model.[12] Culture is assessed from the standpoint of company relationships and management tasks to determine the degree and source of cultural risk.

Allen and Kraft[13] propose a normative systems model with the following four phases:

- discovery
- involving people
- bringing about change
- evaluating and renewing

Key norm influences are identified and altered. Cultural objectives are set along with performance and programmatic objectives. The process is ongoing, self-evaluating, and self-renewing.

Deal and Kennedy call for a diagnostic profile that enables the observer to learn about the culture and predict organizational performance.[14] The process begins at the surface of the company and proceeds inward. They suggest the following steps.

1. Study the physical setting to determine consistency among sites and across employee classes.
2. Read what the company says about its culture in its annual reports and company house organs. By content analysis, track key belief statements over time.
3. Examine how the company greets strangers—note the reception area and the duties and responses of receptionists.
4. Interview company people and look for consensual and conflicting perceptions. Learn about the history of the company (myths). Ask why the company is a success, and what explains its growth (values). Inquire what kind of people work there, and who really gets ahead in the long run (heroes). Ask what kind of place it is to work for, and what an average day is like (rituals).
5. Observe how people spend their time and compare what people say they do to what they actually do (cultural cohesion).

With the data derived from the above observations, determine the present dominant culture and how it has changed over time. Make tentative conclusions as to whether the culture is inwardly or outwardly focused, whether it is strong or weak, or whether it is a focused or fragmented culture. It then may be possible to make preliminary statements about the direction of the firm and its anticipated business strategies.

Typology

Deal and Kennedy,[15] Handy,[16] and Harrison[17] contend that four types of corporate cultures exist. In real life, no company exactly fits any of the four types, but certain attributes usually predominate. Using Deal and Kennedy's[18] terminology, the four types are (Figure 9-1):

1. *The Tough-Guy Macho Culture:* A world of individuals who regularly take high risks and get quick feedback on whether their actions were right (police departments, surgeons, the entertainment industry)
2. *The Work Hard/Play Hard Culture:* Fun and action are the rule here, and employees take few risks with quick feedback; to succeed, the culture encourages them to maintain a high level of low-risk activity (sales organizations, office equipment manufacturers, and all retail stores)
3. *The Bet Your Company Culture:* Cultures with big stakes decisions, where years pass before employees know whether decisions have paid off; a high-risk, slow-feedback environment (capital goods companies, oil companies, and the Army and Navy)

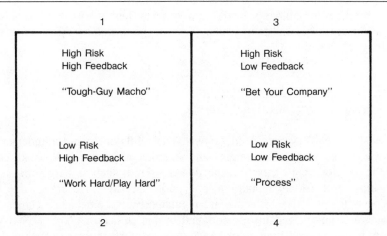

Figure 9-1 A Matrix of Cultural Typology. *Source: Corporate Cultures* by T.E. Deal and A.A. Kennedy, pp. 107–127, Addison-Wesley Publishing Company © 1982.

4. *The Process Culture:* A world of little or no feedback where employees find it hard to measure what they do; instead they concentrate on how it is done (banks, insurance companies, and government)

Companies with strong cultures hardly fit any of these simple modes. These companies have cultures that blend the best elements of all four types and blend them in ways that allow the companies to perform well when the environment around them changes. The biggest single influence on a company's culture is the broader social and business environment in which the company operates.

LEADERSHIP AND THE ORGANIZATIONAL CULTURE

All the authors emphasize leadership in the shaping and management of an organizational culture. Peters and Waterman note that while excellent companies are driven by coherent value systems, all of them are marked by the personality of a leader who laid down the value set.[19] Charismatic personality has little to do with leadership. Instead it comes from obvious, sincere, sustained personal commitment to the values the leaders sought to implant, coupled with extraordinary persistence in reinforcing those values. Persistence and the leader's visibility are vital among excellent companies. Leaders seem to unleash excitement. Clarifying and breathing life into the value system are among the greatest contributions a leader can make. However, creating and instilling a value system isn't easy. Only a few value systems are right for a given company. Instilling a value system is hard work requiring persistence, travel, and long hours. Without this hands-on direct approach, nothing much happens.

Managing the Organizational Culture

Neustadt's book on presidential power is a useful document for understanding the management of a complex and fragmented culture.[20] Neustadt calls for the development of presidential power sources such as bargaining relationships, professional reputation, and public prestige. He argues that the prospects for effective influence are regulated by the president's choices of objectives, timing, and instruments and by his choice of choices to avoid. Peters has examined how chief executives spend their time.[21] Rather than being distressed by the lack of order [in the organization], the executive has many opportunities to manage the company's values and alter its direction.

CHANGING THE ORGANIZATIONAL CULTURE

Once the executive has defined and categorized the corporate culture, these options emerge:

- Ignore the culture.
- Manage around the culture.
- Try to change the culture to fit the strategy.
- Try to change his or her strategy to fit the culture.

If the executive chooses to change the culture, then much work must be done. A major shift in the corporate culture can take anywhere from 3 to 8 years.[22] Management must spend 5–10 percent of its annual budget for the personnel whose behavior is supposed to be changed. To get people in a culture even to begin to change, management has to capture 5–10% of their time for a year.[23]

Cultural change implies real changes in the behavior of people throughout the organization. There will be new heroes, new stories, and new allocations of time. Cultural change[24] is called for when:

- The environment is undergoing fundamental change after the company has always been value driven.
- The industry is highly competitive, and the environment changes quickly.
- The company is mediocre or worse.
- The company is at the threshold of becoming a large organization.
- The company is growing rapidly.

In most other situations, large-scale cultural change should not be undertaken.

Managers contemplating change should focus on the following five factors: consensus, two-way trust, skill building, patience, and flexibility.

In reviewing similarities from case studies of organizational culture change, Ouchi found the following[25]:

- The change initiator was someone who enjoyed a high degree of freedom.

- The organization was in a healthy state when it began the change.
- The leader who initiated the change saw distant early warning signals and decided to take action to forestall trouble.
- The leaders of cultural change had strong moral character.
- Support from the top of the organization was essential for the effort to succeed.

Silverzweig and Allen note common pitfalls in the cultural change process that result in wasted time and money and build unrealistic expectations that exacerbate cynicism, apathy, and frustration.[26]

- lip-service commitment from the Chief Executive Officer
- adherence to traditional win-lose attitudes
- inadequate involvement of all levels of employees
- insufficient attention to middle management
- inappropriate pace of the change effort
- inappropriate level of expectation
- failure to internalize the change process

FUTURE CULTURES

Deal and Kennedy[27] propose that the organization of the future will consist of small task-focused work units (10-20 persons maximum), each with economical and managerial control for its own destiny, interconnected with larger entities through computer and communication links, and bonded into larger companies through strong cultural bonds. They call this structure an "atomized organization" to emphasize the small size and flexibility of its basic units. The company's elements are linked through telecommunication and bonded into a strong corporate whole through shared cultural ties that define the company's future.

Companies that may fare well in the future are McDonald's and the U.S. Forest Service. These are human institutions that capture some expressive aspects of living: soul, spirit, magic, heart, ethos, mission, and saga. The authors conclude that building strong corporate cultures is one of the fundamental management tasks of the next decade. The future holds promise for strong culture companies with an ability to respond to the environment and adapt to diverse and changing circumstances.

STUDIES

Nonhealth Care

Peters and Waterman[28] and Wright[29] offer insights on how corporate cultures can shape business strategies. Pascale and Athos[30] argue that when an American manager wants to make organizational changes, he or she focuses on strategy, structure, and systems—the "hardware" of management science. The Japanese manager, while not ignoring hardware, focuses on the "software"—skills, staff, style, and shared values. The linking device for the hardware and software of management is the shared values of a corporation. This "7-S" framework is useful for management analysis (See Exhibit 9-1 and Figure 9-2.)

Health Care

Marvin Weisbord[31] has compiled data on academic medical centers: "process" cultures marked by the absence of widely accepted organizational performance measures. A review of task conflicts, conflict resolution mechanisms, reporting paths, and reward systems suggests a culture that places high regard on research, subspecialization, and academic freedom. Low regard is given to administrative activities.

In 1976, Money studied organizational behavior in 16 health care systems.[32] Varying organizational perceptions existed between corporate staff and hospital managers, people involved in patient care versus administration, and people higher up in the hierarchy than others. This suggests that the corporate cultures were weak, in transition, and that corporate managers failed to place culture management high on their priority list. Older systems had less uncertainty, tolerated more decentralized decision making, were less

---

Exhibit 9-1 McKinsey 7-S Framework

Structure	Shared Values
Systems	Skills
Style	Strategy
Staff	

Source: In Search of Excellence by T.J. Peters and R.H. Waterman, Jr., p. 10, Harper & Row Publishers, © 1982.

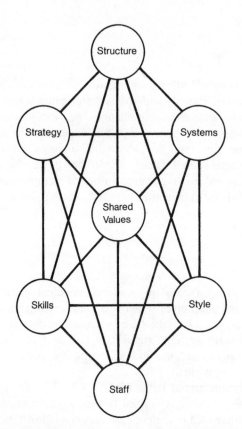

Strategy
Plan or course of action leading to the allocation of a firm's scarce resources, over time, to reach identified goals.

Structure
Characterization of the organization chart (i.e., functional, decentralized, etc.).

Systems
Proceduralized reports and routinized processes such as meeting formats.

Staff
"Demographics" description of important personnel categories within the firm (i.e., engineers, entrepreneurs, M.B.A.s, etc.). "Staff" is not meant in line-staff terms.

Style
Characterization of how key managers behave in achieving the organization's goals; also the cultural style of the organization.

Skills
Distinctive capabilities of key personnel or the firm as a whole.

Shared Values
The significant meanings or guiding concepts that an organization imbues in its members.

Figure 9-2 The Seven Ss. Source: Reprinted from *The Art of Japanese Management: Applications for American Executives* by R.T. Pascale and A.G. Athos, p. 125. Copyright© 1981 by Richard Tanner Pascale and Anthony G. Athos. Reprinted with permission of Simon & Schuster, Inc.

resistant to system goals, and had stronger cultures. The traumas associated with the initiation of systems last from 5 to 10 years. The older the system, the more likely it is that the trauma had been handled and organizational processes have fallen in place.

Health Management Company Cultures

I have studied the corporate cultures of four health management companies to determine dominant culture, typology, and anticipated strategies. Each firm is large and covers a multistate area. All operate in highly competitive environments. Each firm's culture was shaped by a strong leader. Respective cultures have evolved as the organization has grown and prospered. Two of the four organizations have already reorganized, while the other two are seriously considering it. Although each can be viewed as a major system, there is room for further growth, development, and linkages with other systems (Table 9-1).

Table 9-1 Health Management Company

Feature	A	B	C	D
A. Cultural Dimensions				
Inward/Outward	Inward	Outward	Inward	Outward
Strong/Weak	Weak in transition	Strongest at corporate level	Strong, but shifting	Strongest at corporate level
Focused/ Fragmented	Fragmented + +	Fragmented +	Fragmented + + +	Fragmented +
Innovation: Leader/Follower	Follower	Leader	Follower	Leader
Market Approach: Aggressive/ Conservative	Conservative, but shifting	Aggressive!	Conservative	Aggressive
Future Orientation: Growth/ Survival	Survival, but shifting	Growth	Survival	Growth
B. Typology	Process	Work hard/play hard	Process	Bet Your Company
C. Anticipated Strategies and Issues	Old and new values clash	Shedding old business lines	New corporate staff and value conflicts	Acquire or merge
	Complete transition	Rapid growth in new ventures	Move to centralize	Difficult leadership transition
	Moderate, staggered growth in short term	Need to assimilate changes	Difficult leadership transition	Complex organizational to structures
	Slow change process	Newer values predominate	Status quo regarding reorganization	Additional reorganization to follow
	Reorganization will occur, possibly "bottom up"	Additional reorganization to follow	Moderate, fairly constant growth rate	Sporadic, but significant growth when it occurs

APPLICATION STRATEGIES

The Lutheran Hospitals and Homes Society is one of the nation's oldest and largest not-for-profit multi-unit providers. It owns, leases, and manages 82 facilities in 14 states, from Alaska to Arizona. Most units are in rural areas, adding to the problem of geographical dispersion. Historically, a strong culture helped to bind the various units into a coherent whole. Today, environmental demands have placed a premium on implementation of management "hardware"—strategies, structure, and systems. Ironically, the need for a shared value system has never been greater. This revised culture must be contemporary, but still reinforce the historical values and beliefs that have made the Society strong. The system's COO has made a multiyear commitment to cultural change and views the management of culture as one of the key tasks.

To be successful, a management undertaking must be supported by top officials with recognition and acceptance of culture management as a useful tool. A study of the literature is a necessary first step. Use of consultants may also be advisable. With an understanding of culture management must also come an acceptance of the time and resource commitment. The tasks cannot be easily delegated, and emphasis must be on action, rather than words. Top management must embody the key values of the culture and reinforce them in everything it does.

Any evaluation of a corporate culture should begin with an assessment of the existing management philosophy. Comparing actual performance with the company's mission statement presents the "goodness of fit" between the statement and the day-to-day functioning of the organization. Such an examination could alter, reinforce, or change the underlying philosophy.

Once you make the decision to change your corporate culture, you can choose interventions. Weigh each intervention carefully, looking for opportunities, such as environmental issues like competition, or financial shortfalls, or personnel changes, including retirement.

- *Recruitment*—Alter your requirements or broaden your search to locate people who might better fit the revised culture.
- *Orientation*—Make deliberate attempts to socialize new recruits into the altered culture.
- *Management development efforts*—Design continuing education programs so that the values and beliefs of the new culture are explained and strengthened.

- *Performance appraisal*—Redesign overall corporate measures, such as critical success factors, to emphasize desired changes in the culture. Individual performance appraisals should stress achievement of tasks that reinforce the desired cultural change.
- *Reorganization/reassignment*—Redefine duties and responsibilities and alter reporting paths to change the culture.
- *Innovation audit*—With the assistance of outside consultants, conduct an innovation audit to assess the degree of innovation within the organization, identify cultural barriers that stifle innovation, and suggest strategies for improving the innovative environment.

Hardly unique to culture management, these interventions are straightforward management strategies. In this instance, they are used to achieve cultural objectives.

There are lower-cost alternatives to achieving cultural changes.[33]

- Develop a statement of corporate purpose, list the company beliefs, and remind everyone about it.
- Tailor your formal systems, structures, and personnel policies to reflect the company beliefs.

Find out whether it's more courageous to take action now or defer action until the corporate culture has been appropriately transformed. Set *modest* goals for cultural change. It is a long, difficult process, and short-term wholesale change won't occur.

SUMMARY

Irreversible societal trends indicate that hospitals and health management companies must restructure, reorganize, and reconceptualize their businesses. This implies a "sea change" in the way health care is now provided. But first this massive strategical shift must be preceded by an analysis of the company's culture and an effort to reshape the culture so that such changes are supported throughout the organization. Many health care executives are open to organizational change, but incapable of dealing with the underlying culture that must occur. How managers identify, manage, and redirect their respective cultures is crucial. It's a difficult, costly, time-consuming effort, but essential if sustained change is to be achieved.

140   STRATEGIC MANAGEMENT

NOTES

1. John Naisbitt, *Megatrends* (New York: Warner Books, 1982), chapter 5.

2. Robert Reich, "The Next American Frontier," *The Atlantic,* March 1983, 43–58.

3. W.G. Ouchi, *Theory Z* (New York: Avon Books, 1981), 111–191.

4. M. Maccoby, *The Leader* (New York: Simon and Schuster, 1981), 191.

5. H. Schwartz and S.M. Davis, "Matching Corporate Culture and Business Strategy," *Organizational Dynamics,* Summer 1981, 30–48.

6. R.F. Allen and C. Kraft, "Discovering Your Hospital's Unconscious," *Hospital Forum* January/February 1983, 12.

7. T.E. Deal and A.A. Kennedy, *Corporate Cultures* (Reading, MA: Addison-Wesley Publishing Company, 1982), 3–19.

8. Chester Barnard, *The Functions of the Executive* (Cambridge: Harvard University Press, 1938), 79–87.

9. Philip Selznick, *Leadership in Administration* (New York, Harper and Row, 1957), 28.

10. T.E. Deal, A.A. Kennedy, and A.H. Spiegel III, "How to Create an Outstanding Hospital Culture," *Hospital Forum,* January/February 1983, 22–24.

11. Ibid, 24–25.

12. H. Schwartz and S.M. Davis, op. cit., pp. 30–48.

13. R.F. Allen and C. Kraft, op. cit., 15–19.

14. T.E. Deal and A.A. Kennedy, op. cit., 129–139.

15. Ibid, 107–127.

16. C.B. Handy, *Understanding Organizations,* second edition, (Middlesex, England: Penguin Books Ltd., 1981), 177–185.

17. R. Harrison, "Understanding Your Organization's Character," *Harvard Business Review,* May-June 1972, 121–123.

18. T.E. Deal and A.A. Kennedy, op. cit., 107–127.

19. T.J. Peters and R.H. Waterman Jr., *In Search of Excellence* (New York: Harper and Row, 1982), 279–291.

20. R.E. Neustadt, *Presidential Power* (New York: John Wiley and Sons, 1980), chapters 5 and 6.

21. T.J. Peters, "Leadership: Sad Facts and Silver Linings," *Harvard Business Review,* November-December 1979, 164–172.

22. Ibid, p. 170.

23. T.E. Deal and A.A. Kennedy, op. cit., 161–162.

24. Ibid, 159–166.

25. W.G. Ouchi, op. cit., 163–164.

26. R.A. Silverzweig and R.F. Allen, "Changing the Corporate Culture," *Sloan Management Review,* Spring 1976, 47–48.

27. T.E. Deal and A.A. Kennedy, op. cit., 177–196.

28. T.J. Peters and R.H. Waterman, Jr., op. cit., chapter 6.

29. J.P. Wright, *On a Clear Day You Can See General Motors* (New York: Warner Books, 1981), 126–135.

30. R.T. Pascale and A.G. Athos, *The Art of Japanese Management* (New York: Warner Books, 1981), 58–84.

31. M.R. Weisbord, "Three Dilemmas of Academic Medical Centers," *Journal of Applied Behavioral Science,* 14, no. 3 (1978):284–304.

32. W.H. Money, et al., "A Comparative Study of Multi-Unit Health Care Organizations," in *Organizational Research in Hospitals,* ed. S.M. Shortell and M. Brown (Chicago: Inquiry, 1976), 29–61.

33. Bro Uttal, "The Corporate Culture Vultures," *Fortune,* October 17, 1983, 66–72.

Matrix Analysis Techniques for Strategic Business Units

Two matrix analysis techniques can be applied to the analysis of strategic business units (SBUs) in health care corporations: the growth share matrix (GSM) and the service area attractiveness-SBU business strength (SAASBS) matrix. The concept of a SBU is used by nearly all large industrial corporations to identify those organizational units within the corporation that can be viewed as relatively autonomous. The SBU usually has its own president and always has its own general manager. Often, the SBU is a separate corporation; it is always a separate corporate entity that has its own financial reports and can be viewed as a profit center.

In Chapter 10 the growth share matrix is described in detail as it applies to strategic business units (SBUs) in a health care setting.

Chapter 11 discusses the service area attractiveness-SBU business strength (SAASBS) matrix analysis technique. Especially for evaluating SBUs, the SAASBS matrix analysis technique is far superior than the growth share matrix analysis technique, which only measures service area growth rate of the particular service provided by the SBU and relative market share of the SBU in the service area.

The last chapter in this part, Chapter 12, uses a case study of a multi-institutional health care organization to illustrate the application of both the growth share matrix analysis technique and the SAASBS matrix analysis technique.

Strategic Business Unit Analysis with the Growth Share Matrix

Chapter 10

Strategic Business Unit
Analysis with the
Growth Share Matrix

HIGHLIGHTS

- Plotting the Growth Share Matrix
- Illustration of the Growth Share Matrix
- Summary

10

The primary use of the growth share matrix (GSM) is as a tool to evaluate strategic business units (SBUs) of larger corporations, such as multihospital corporations, multi-HMO corporations, multinursing home corporations, and combinations of the above. Exhibit 10-1 lists examples of SBUs in health care corporations.

The growth share matrix as used for SBUs has been well publicized by the popular business press because of its designation of SBUs by such names as stars, cash cows, dogs, and problem children.

PLOTTING THE GROWTH SHARE MATRIX

The growth share matrix is shown in Figure 10-1. The vertical axis measures the annual growth rate of the strategic business unit (SBU) of the health care corporation in the service area covered by the SBU. The horizontal axis measures the relative market share of each SBU in the respective service area. Relative market share is determined by dividing the health care corporation's SBU market share by the market share of the leading competitor. If the SBU has the largest market share, then the competitor having the next largest market share is defined as the leading competitor.

In Figure 10-1, note that the range of relative market share runs from 0.1 to 1.5 with the dividing line at 0.8. The relative market share figures in this case are arbitrarily selected. However, in real world applications relative market share depends on the particular organization, the competitiveness in the service area, and the diversity of the SBUs. If possible all SBUs should be plottable within the confines of the selected dimensions. If this is not feasible, a SBU can, of course, always be shown with an asterisk and footnote at the left or right extreme boundary line, whichever is appropriate.

Exhibit 10-1 Examples of Strategic Business Units in Typical Health Care Organizations

Cameron Hospital
Sonoma Hospital
Sheridan Hospital
Tonawanda Nursing Home
Bluebird Nursing Home
Frontier Health Maintenance Organization
Regional Home Health Care Corporation
Youngstown Ambulatory Care Center
Willowdale Ambulatory Health Care Center
Riverside Ambulatory Health Care Center
Wheatfield Preferred Provider Organization
Niagara Urgent Care Centers
Physicians Health Insurance

Similarly, the annual service area growth rates plotted on the vertical axis are selected so that all SBUs can be plotted on the matrix. In Figure 10-1 service area growth rates range from 0 to 12 percent, with the bisecting line at 6 percent. If a SBU with an extremely high growth rate that causes it to go off the scale needs to be plotted, it can, of course, be located at the upper boundary line. Similarly, a SBU with a negative growth rate can be plotted

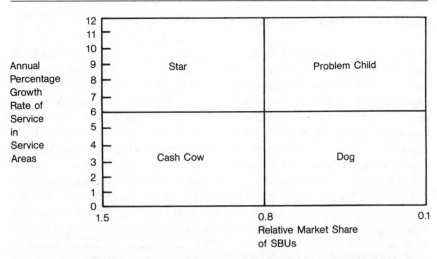

Note: Relative market share is the ratio of corporation's SBU market share to leading competitor market share. If the corporation's SBU has the largest market share, then the leading competitor is the SBU with the next highest market share.

Figure 10-1 Growth Share Matrix of Strategic Business Units

near the bottom boundary line. In both cases the SBUs should be identified with an asterisk and footnote.

Both the relative market share and annual percentage growth rate dimensions and division lines should be selected so that the various SBUs of the corporation can be located across the entire matrix. In other words, the growth share matrix would not reveal very much if all SBUs were located in a single cell; say, the upper right hand cell of the matrix.

Note that the four cells have been identified by the names of star, cash cow, problem child, and dog. The appropriateness of these names has been and is still under debate, and the criticism of the names is quite valid. In numerous instances so-called dog SBUs have been very successful, and many so-called stars have fallen and failed. However, these names are used here because of common industry practice. The reader may want to use other names or not use names at all.

ILLUSTRATION OF THE GROWTH SHARE MATRIX

The use of the growth share matrix can best be illustrated with a case example. Suppose that the corporation to which the growth share matrix is applied is Eastern Medical Enterprises (EME). EME owns four hospitals in four nonoverlapping service areas, three nursing homes also in nonoverlapping service areas, and one home health care organization.

Each one of the four hospitals, the three nursing homes, and the home health care organization is considered a SBU. The growth rates, market shares, and leading competitor market shares for each of the eight SBUs are shown in Table 10-1. Note that hospital A has the largest market share, 45 percent, in its respective service area. The market shares of the three other hospitals are 40 percent, 30 percent, and 20 percent, respectively. Nursing homes typically serve larger service areas than hospitals, and as a result the market shares of the three nursing homes are 18 percent, 15 percent, and 10 percent, respectively. The home health care organization is the market share leader in its respective service area and commands 50 percent of the market.

The service area growth rates range from a low of 2 percent for hospital C to a high of 7 percent for nursing home BB. The leading competitor market shares in the respective service areas produce relative market shares ranging from a low of 0.5 for hospital D to a high of 2.8 for the home health care organization.

All eight SBUs are plotted on the growth share matrix shown on Figure 10-2. Note that the relative market share axis ranges from 0 to 3.0, with the bisecting line at 1.5. The annual percentage growth rate axis ranges from 0 to 9 percent, with the bisecting line at 4.5 percent.

Table 10-1 Summary of SBU Market Shares, Leading Competitor Market Shares, Relative Market Shares, and Service Area Growth Rates: Eastern Medical Enterprises

SBU	Service Area Growth Rate (%)	SBU Market Share (%)	Leading Competitor Market Share (%)	Relative Market Share
Hospital A	4	45	25	1.8
Hospital B	6	40	20	2.0
Hospital C	2	30	50	0.6
Hospital D	3	20	40	0.5
Nursing Home AA	4	18	20	0.9
Nursing Home BB	7	15	8	1.9
Nursing Home CC	5	10	9	1.1
Home Health Care Organization AAA	6	50	18	2.8

Note: Relative market share is the ratio of corporation's SBU market share to the leading competitor's market share. If the corporation's SBU has the largest market share, then the leading competitor is the SBU with the next highest market share.

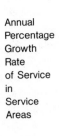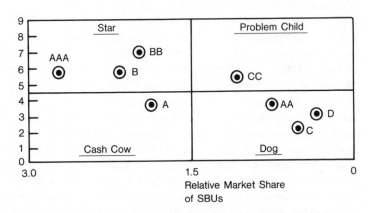

Note: Relative market share is the ratio of EME's SBU market share to the leading competitor market share.

A, B, C, D—hospitals A, B, C, and D
AA, BB, CC—nursing homes AA, BB, and CC
AAA—home health care organization

Figure 10-2 Growth Share Matrix: Eastern Medical Enterprises

After plotting the eight SBUs on the growth share matrix, three SBUs fall in the upper left hand cell of the matrix, the cell that is designated as "star." Hence, three of the eight SBUs—hospital B, nursing home BB, and the home health care organization—are stars. Hospital A falls in the "cash cow" cell and three SBUs—hospitals C and D and nursing home AA—fall in the "dog" cell. Finally, one SBU, nursing home CC, falls in the "problem child" cell. Therefore, the eight SBUs are reasonably well distributed over the four cells of the growth share matrix.

The three SBUs in the "dog" cell of the matrix have growth rates in the respective service areas that are quite low, from 2 to 4 percent, and relative market shares that are quite low, from 0.5 to 0.9. Actual market shares range from 18 to 30 percent. It is of course possible that market shares could increase, especially for the nursing home. However, it will be probably difficult to increase the market shares for hospitals C and D because of the relatively slow service area growth rate and the difficulties that hospitals face in increasing market share significantly in low growth service areas. The two "dog" hospitals, hospitals C and D, are therefore somewhat undesirable properties for future growth of EME. If divestment is an option, EME should probably consider it for C and D and invest the proceeds in health care properties in more promising areas. It is, of course, possible that hospitals C and D are good cash cows. In that case they should be retained and used to generate cash for the expansion of the "star" SBUs.

Whether these assigned designations for the SBUs are correct is of course up for debate. Remember that the growth share matrix only considers relative market share and SBU growth rate; no consideration is given to profitability.

SUMMARY

In this chapter the SBU growth share matrix was applied to the example of Eastern Medical Enterprises, which has eight SBUs. The matrix was constructed so that it satisfied the parameters of each of the eight SBUs.

It is important to recognize the limitations of the growth share matrix. It only measures relative market share and SBU growth rate in the service area. Hence, no information is collected on profitability, cash flows, or compatibility with other SBUs. Nevertheless, the growth share matrix has been popular over the years and still remains popular because it is relatively easy to apply, requires data that are relatively widely available, and produces results that are, at least at first glance, easy to understand.

The next chapter discusses an alternative to the growth share matrix. It is more difficult and time consuming to apply but it produces more useful results.

Strategic Business Unit Evaluation with Service Area Attractiveness-SBU Business Strength Matrix

Strategic Analysis and
Evaluation with Service Area
Attractiveness-SBU Business
Strength Matrix

HIGHLIGHTS

- Service Area Attractiveness-SBU Business Strength Matrix
- Illustration of the Service Area Attractiveness-SBU Business Strength Matrix
- Summary

11

The development of the service area attractiveness-SBU business strength (SAASBS) matrix is generally attributed to the General Electric Corporation, which presumably used it first because it found the growth share matrix to be somewhat limited. The SAASBS matrix, as was the growth share matrix, was developed for the purpose of evaluating SBUs of larger corporations.

The growth share matrix presented in Chapter 10 has been highly publicized in the popular business press because of its dog, cash cow, star, and problem child designations. The SAASBS matrix, in contrast, is relatively unknown and has been treated with benign neglect by the popular business press. However, it is more useful for evaluation and analysis purposes and is quite widely used by organizations with active strategic planning programs.

This chapter discusses the application of the SAASBS matrix to strategic business units (SBUs) of health care service corporations. As previously mentioned, strategic business units of large health care service corporations can have a variety of organizational formats. A quite common one is the self-standing community or specialty hospital owned by the health care service corporation. Other types of SBUs are nursing homes, home health care organizations, ambulatory health centers, surgical centers, and self-standing emergency centers.

SERVICE AREA ATTRACTIVENESS-SBU BUSINESS
STRENGTH MATRIX

The framework of a typical service area attractiveness-SBU business strength matrix is shown in Figure 11-1. The vertical axis measures the SBU business strength in the respective service area, and the horizontal axis measures the attractiveness of the respective service segment in the service area. Note that the axes are measured on a 2.0 to 3.5 scale. This scale is used

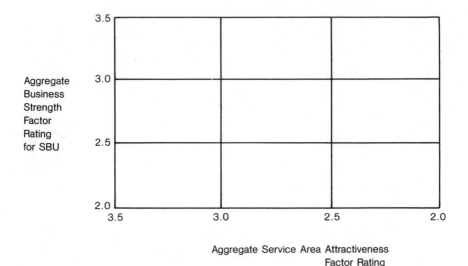

Aggregate Business Strength Factor Rating for SBU

Aggregate Service Area Attractiveness
Factor Rating

Figure 11-1 A Typical Service Area Attractiveness-SBU Business Strength Matrix

because the various factors that determine the SBU business strength or the service area attractiveness are measured on a 1 to 4 scale, where the scale ranges from poor (1) to strong (4) for SBU business strength and from unattractive (1) to attractive (4) for the service area. Because almost any factor will at least receive some positive evaluation, the actual range of the aggregated factors falls commonly in the 2.0 to 3.5 range.

Examples of SBU business strength factors are financial, marketing, quality of services, and accessibility; examples of service area attractiveness are growth rate, profitability, ease of entry, and competitiveness. Each one of the factors is assigned a rating between 1 and 4, and each is weighted. The weighted ratings are then combined into an overall measure of SBU business strength and service area attractiveness.

Table 11-1 shows how ratings and weights are combined for the business strength component; the aggregation of service area attractiveness factors for a SBU is shown in Table 11-2. Note that in all cases the weights applied to the factors must add up to 1.00 in order to obtain an unbiased aggregate rating.

In the case of the service area attractiveness factors, a factor, such as ease of entry, is given a low value of 1 if it is easy to enter that particular service area for a new organization; conversely, a high value of 4 is assigned if it is very difficult to enter that particular service area. If ease of entry is high, then more competitors are bound to enter and thus make the service area less attractive. Competitiveness is given a low value of 1 if there is strong compe-

Table 11-1 Aggregation of SBU Business Strength Factor Ratings: SBU Evaluation

Business Strength Factors for SBU	Rating	Weight	Rating × Weight
Financial	2.4	.20	.48
Marketing	1.6	.15	.24
Quality of services	2.8	.25	.70
Accessibility	2.7	.20	.54
Staff competence	3.1	.20	.62
Aggregate rating		1.00	2.58

tition and a high value of 4 if competition is weak. As above, weak competition enhances the attractiveness of the service area.

ILLUSTRATION OF THE SERVICE AREA ATTRACTIVENESS-SBU BUSINESS STRENGTH MATRIX

Continuing the example discussed in Chapter 10, the SAASBS matrix is applied to Eastern Medical Enterprises Corporation (EME), a health care concern made up of eight SBUs—four hospitals, three nursing homes, and one home health care organization. Each of the eight SBUs is located in a different service area.

For each of the eight SBUs, senior management developed aggregate service area attractiveness factor ratings and aggregate SBU business strength factor ratings. The service area attractiveness factors that management identified, which were the same for all eight SBUs, were service area growth rate for the particular health service segment, profitability of the health service in the service area, ease of entry for that particular health service in the service area, competitiveness of the health service in the service area, and government regulations affecting the particular health service in the service area.

Table 11-3 illustrates the aggregate service area attractiveness ratings for one SBU, a nursing home. Note that the nursing home growth rate in the

Table 11-2 Aggregation of Service Segment Attractiveness Factor Ratings: SBU Evaluation

Service Area Attractiveness Factors	Rating	Weight	Rating × Weight
Growth rate	2.5	0.40	1.00
Profitability	2.0	0.20	0.40
Ease of entry	1.8	0.30	0.54
Competitiveness	2.4	0.10	0.24
Aggregate rating		1.00	2.18

Table 11-3 Aggregation of Service Area Attractiveness Factor Ratings: Nursing Home

Factors for Health Service	Rating	Weight	Rating × Weight
Growth rate	3.0	.25	.75
Profitability	2.0	.30	.60
Ease of entry	3.0	.10	.30
Competitiveness	2.5	.10	.25
Regulation effects	1.5	.25	.38
Aggregate rating		1.00	2.28

service area being served by the nursing home is quite strong. As a result, a rating of 3.0 for the health service growth rate in the respective service area has been assigned. This procedure to determine the service area attractiveness factor ratings was repeated for each of the other seven SBUs.

The next step is to determine aggregate SBU business strength factor ratings for each of the eight SBUs. Senior management identified five SBU business strength factors that it wanted to use to determine the aggregate SBU business strength factor rating for each of the eight SBUs. The five SBU business strength factors were financial, marketing, quality of services, accessibility, and staff competence.

Table 11-4 illustrates how senior management determined the aggregate SBU business strength factor rating for home health care services. Note that one of the business strengths of EME's home health care organization was accessibility because the home health care organization was located in the center of a relatively older population whose need for home health care was quite high. The other SBU business strengths were quality of services and staff competence. Its extensive experience and good reputation in patient care delivery enabled the home health care unit to attract high quality personnel, which, in turn, contributed greatly to these two SBU business strengths of quality of services and staff competence.

Table 11-4 Aggregation of SBU Business Strength Factor Ratings: Home Health Care Organization

Factors for SBU Strength	Rating	Weight	Rating × Weight
Financial	2.5	.20	.50
Marketing	2.5	.20	.50
Quality of services	3.4	.25	.85
Accessibility	3.5	.10	.35
Staff competence	3.6	.25	.90
Aggregate rating		1.00	3.10

The above procedure to determine the aggregate SBU business strength factor rating for home health care services was repeated for the other seven SBUs. The results are shown in Table 11-5 and include both the aggregate SBU business strength factor ratings and the aggregate service area attractiveness factor ratings for all eight SBUs.

The next step in the SBU analysis evaluation using the SAASBS matrix approach is to plot each of the eight SBUs on the SAASBS matrix, as shown in Figure 11-2. In the SAASBS matrix, as well as in the growth share matrix discussed in Chapter 10, the most desirable SBUs appear in the upper left corner of the matrix. Conversely, the least desirable SBUs appear in the lower right corner of the matrix. Note that the SBU with the highest aggregate factor ratings for both SBU business strength and service area attractiveness is the nursing home (CC), which is in the upper left corner. Not a single SBU fell in the lower right corner of the SAASBS matrix.

In general SBUs falling in the upper left triangle of the SAASBS matrix are quite attractive and usually have a promising future as profit and growth contributors to the organization. SBUs falling in the lower right triangle of the SAASBS matrix are usually potential problems. In some cases they may be resuscitated by management action. However, especially if the aggregate SBU attractiveness factor rating is low, senior management may not have much influence on improving the overall SAASBS matrix status of the SBU.

One can see that EME's SBUs are doing quite well. Only two SBUs are in the lower right triangle of the SAASBS matrix, two are close to the borderline separating the two triangles, and four SBUs are clearly located in the upper left triangle of the SAASBS matrix.

Table 11-5 Aggregate Factor Ratings for Service Area Attractiveness and SBU Business Strength

SBU	Aggregate Service Area Attractiveness Factor Rating	Aggregate SBU Business Strength Factor Rating
Hospital		
A	2.65	2.90
B	2.38	3.06
C	3.14	2.78
D	2.46	2.32
Nursing home		
AA	2.28	2.85
BB	2.38	2.60
CC	3.15	3.20
Home health care organization		
AAA	2.80	3.10

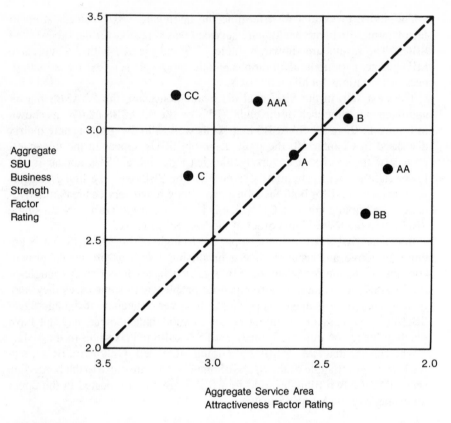

Figure 11-2 Service Area Attractiveness-SBU Business Strength Matrix: Eastern Medical Enterprises

---

SUMMARY

In this chapter the service area attractiveness-SBU business strength matrix was applied to a health network corporation with eight SBUs. The SAASBS matrix was constructed so that it fit the parameters of each of the eight SBUs.

Although the SAASBS approach has limitations, it evaluates SBUs in a much more comprehensive manner than the growth share matrix discussed in Chapter 10. Whereas the growth share matrix largely measures SBU market share and service area growth rate, the SAASBS also measures several dimensions of SBU business strength and service area attractiveness: financial, marketing, staff competence, accessibility, and quality of services delivered. Service area attractiveness is measured in terms of growth rate, profitability, ease of entry, competitiveness, and regulation effects.

The disadvantage of the SAASBS matrix in comparison with the growth share matrix is the added work involved in evaluating the various factors that determine SBU business strength and service area attractiveness. However, the work involved in evaluating all factors will provide senior management with a deeper and more extensive knowledge of the factors that determine whether a SBU is a poor or good performer. The extensive evaluation and analysis also determine whether a SBU should receive particular attention and resources from the corporation because of the promise it shows in the strategic plan of the corporation.

Chapter 12

Case Illustration of the Growth Share Matrix and the Service Area Attractiveness-SBU Business Strength Matrix

HIGHLIGHTS

- Description of Delaware Ambulatory Health Care Centers
- Application of the Growth Share Matrix to Delaware Ambulatory Health Care Centers
- Application of the Service Area Attractiveness-SBU Business Strength Matrix to Delaware Ambulatory Health Care Centers
- Summary

12

DESCRIPTION OF DELAWARE AMBULATORY HEALTH CARE CENTERS

Delaware Ambulatory Health Care Centers operates three ambulatory health care centers in the communities of Youngstown, Riverside, and Willowdale. The communities are all small cities or towns in a Midwestern state. Youngstown has a population of about 30,000 people, but is adjacent to a larger urban area. Riverside has a population of about 40,000 and is relatively isolated. The nearest population center is 30 miles away. Willowdale is a suburb of a larger urban area. Willowdale has a population of about 35,000 people.

Each one of the ambulatory care centers competes with other ambulatory care centers and with solo practitioners. However, in each case the Delaware Ambulatory Care Center has the highest market share in the service area covered.

A detailed evaluation of the three ambulatory care centers revealed that there was considerable variability among them in terms of marketing, staff stability, accessibility, quality of services, and financial position (Table 12-1). The Youngstown center has an extensive marketing program, but its staffing is weaker because of its higher rates of absenteeism and staff turnover. The Youngstown center also has the easiest access of the three centers. It is located on a main bus line, and a bus stop is located in front of its door. In addition, it has excellent parking facilities and is located close to an expressway. The other two centers have relatively poorer accessibility at their locations.

The Youngstown ambulatory care center has the strongest financial position of the three. It has excellent financial and operating ratios and generates the highest gross margin on revenues.

Table 12-1 Summary of Several Factors of Each Strategic Business Unit (SBU)

SBU Business Strength Factor	Youngstown Center	Riverside Center	Willowdale Center
Market share	24%	20%	16%
Market share of leading competitor	12%	16%	8%
Marketing	Excellent	Good	Very good
Quality of services	Good	Very good	Very good
Staff stability	Weak	Good	Excellent
Accessibility	Excellent	Good	Weak
Financial status	Excellent	Very good	Good

The service areas served by the three ambulatory care centers vary considerably in terms of annual growth rate, competitiveness, and profitability. In the Willowdale market, which has a rapid growth rate, competition is moderate and so far comes largely from solo practitioners. Riverside, with the smallest growth rate, has the most extensive competition. Another ambulatory care center that is somewhat smaller than Riverside is quite aggressive and is attempting to overtake the Delaware center in terms of market share. The Youngstown ambulatory care center has a moderate growth rate and moderate competition. As a result it is an attractive market for possible expansion. Table 12-2 summarizes the factors discussed above.

The vice-president of planning for Delaware Ambulatory Care Centers, James Wallace, decided to evaluate and analyze the three ambulatory care centers using the growth share matrix and the service area attractiveness-SBU business strength matrix. In this analysis he viewed each one of the three ambulatory care centers as a separate strategic business unit (SBU).

APPLICATION OF THE GROWTH SHARE MATRIX TO DELAWARE AMBULATORY HEALTH CARE CENTERS

The growth share matrix is based on just two factors: relative market share and service area annual growth rate for the particular service being considered.

Table 12-2 Factor Evaluation for the Three Service Areas

Service Area	Service Area Annual Growth Rate for Ambulatory Care Services	Competitiveness of Ambulatory Care in Service Area	Profitability of Ambulatory Care Services in Service Area
Youngstown	6%	Moderate	Very good
Riverside	2%	Extensive	Weak
Willowdale	9%	Moderate	Excellent

For each particular ambulatory care center the relative market share can be derived from the market share data in Table 12-1. The calculations to determine relative market share for each ambulatory care center, as well as market share data, are shown in Table 12-3. Note that the Youngstown Center has the highest relative market share, closely followed by the Willowdale Center. The Riverside Center's relative market share is a distant third.

Using the above relative market share data for each ambulatory care center, as well as the service area growth rates shown in Table 12-2, the location of each ambulatory care center can now be plotted on the growth share matrix (Figure 12-1). Note that Willowdale falls in the "star" category, Youngstown falls in the "cash cow" cell but is close to the "star" cell, and Riverside is labeled a "dog." Especially in this case, be cautious about accepting the designations of star, cash cow, and dog. No financial information is presented on Youngstown so how can it be labeled a cash cow? This application of the growth share matrix clearly shows its limitations.

APPLICATION OF THE SERVICE AREA ATTRACTIVENESS-SBU BUSINESS STRENGTH MATRIX TO DELAWARE AMBULATORY HEALTH CARE CENTERS

The first step in applying this matrix to the three health care centers is to develop the SBU business strength aggregate factor. It consists of five subsidiary factors: marketing, quality of services, staff stability, accessibility, and financial status. Table 12-1 lists the evaluations of each of these five factors in terms of nonquantitative descriptions, such as weak, good, very good, and excellent. Now a quantitative numerical rating is applied to each of these nonquantitative descriptions. To the term "weak" is assigned a numerical value of 1, and to the term "good" is assigned a value of 2. A value of 3 is assigned to "very good," and a value of 4 is assigned to "excellent."

Next weights are assigned to each of the five SBU business strength factors. It is, of course, possible to give each factor an equal weight. In the case of Delaware ambulatory care centers, however, that was not the management assessment. The assigned weights vary from a low of 0.10 to a high of 0.30.

Table 12-3 Summary of SBU Relative Market Share for Ambulatory Care Centers

Strategic Business Unit	SBU Market Share	Leading Competitor Market Share	Relative Market Share
Youngstown Center	24	10	2.4
Riverside Center	20	16	1.25
Willowdale Center	16	8	2.0

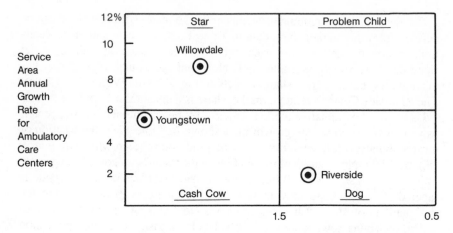

Figure 12-1 Growth Share Matrix for the Three Delaware Ambulatory Health Care Centers

Combining the SBU business strength factor ratings and weights produces an aggregate value for the SAASBS matrix. Table 12-4 shows how the aggregate SBU business strength factor value was determined.

Next the aggregate service area attractiveness factors are determined for the three service areas served by the three Delaware ambulatory health care centers. The aggregate service area attractiveness factor is based on three factors: service area annual growth rate, competitiveness of ambulatory health care centers in the respective service area, and profitability of ambulatory care services in the respective service area. Quantitative estimates are available for the annual growth of ambulatory care services in the service areas. Descriptive evaluations are available for the competitiveness and profitability factors. They are all shown in Table 12-2.

Using the above data the information is translated into quantitative ratings of the three factors. The annual growth ratings are assigned a rating of 1 for an annual growth of 2 percent or less, a rating of 2 for 3–5 percent, a rating of 3 for 6–8 percent, and a rating of 4 for 9 percent and higher. For the descriptive evaluations a rating of 1 is assigned to weak profitability, a rating of 2 to good profitability, a rating of 3 to very good profitability, and a rating of 4 to excellent profitability. Similarly, a rating of 1 is assigned to extensive competitiveness and a rating of 3 to moderate competitiveness. The weights to be assigned to the three service area attractiveness factors are 0.20 for annual growth rate, 0.30 for competitiveness, and 0.50 for profitability.

The aggregate service area attractiveness factor ratings are now determined

Case Illustration   169

Table 12-4 Determination of Aggregate SBU Business Strength Factor Rating for Three SBUs

Center	SBU Business Strength Factor Rating			Weight of Factor			Rating × Weight		
	Y	R	W	Y	R	W	Y	R	W
Business strength factor									
Marketing	4			.10			.40		
		2			.10			.20	
			3			.10			.30
Quality of services	2			.25			.50		
		3			.25			.75	
			3			.25			.75
Staff stability	1			.15			.15		
		2			.15			.30	
			4			.15			.60
Accessibility	4			.20			.80		
		2			.20			.40	
			1			.20			.20
Financial status	4			.30			1.20		
		3			.30			.90	
			2			.30			.60
Aggregate rating of business strength factor							3.05	2.55	2.45

Note: Y = Youngstown
R = Riverside
W = Willowdale

for the three locations where the ambulatory health care centers are located. The method of determination is shown on Table 12-5.

The aggregate service area attractiveness factor ratings are 3.00 for Youngstown, 1.00 for Riverside, and 3.70 for Willowdale. The aggregate service area attractiveness factor ratings and the aggregate SBU business strength factor ratings are plotted on the SAASBS matrix as shown on Figure 12-2.

As can be seen from the SAASBS matrix the same two ambulatory health care centers, Willowdale and Youngstown, that appeared in the upper left triangle of the growth share matrix also appear in the upper left triangle of the SAASBS matrix. The other ambulatory care center, Riverside, is in the lower right cell of the growth share matrix and very close to the lower right cell of the SAASBS matrix.

The only major difference between the two centers—Willowdale and Youngstown—is their appearance in opposite directions on the vertical axes of the growth share matrix and the SAASBS matrix.

Table 12-5 Determination of Aggregate Service Area Attractiveness Factor Ratings for Three Locations

Center	SBU Business Attractiveness Factor Rating			Weight of Factor			Rating × Weight		
	Y	R	W	Y	R	W	Y	R	W
Service area attractiveness factor									
Annual growth rate	3			0.20			0.60		
		1			0.20			0.20	
			4			0.20			0.80
Competitiveness	3			0.30			0.90		
		1			0.30			0.30	
			3			0.30			0.90
Profitability	3			0.50			1.50		
		1			0.50			0.50	
			4			0.50			2.00
Aggregate rating of service area attractiveness factor							3.00	1.00	3.70

Note: Y = Youngstown
R = Riverside
W = Willowdale

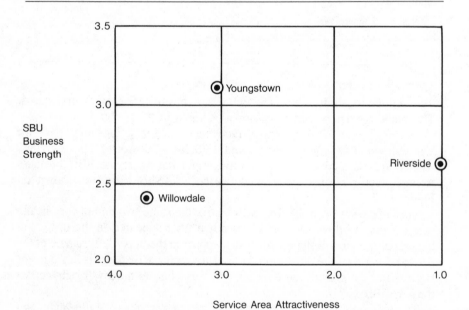

Figure 12-2 Service Area Attractiveness-SBU Business Strength Matrix for the Three Delaware Ambulatory Health Care Centers

SUMMARY

This illustrated in detail how one can position strategic business units, such as three ambulatory health care centers located in three different locations, onto the growth share matrix and the service area attractiveness-SBU business strength matrix.

The approach used converts either quantitative measures, such as annual growth rates, or nonquantitative and descriptive indicators into quantitative factor ratings. Also described was the method used to derive an aggregate factor rating for both SBU business strength and service area attractiveness. This aggregate factor rating was obtained by assigning weights to each of the separate factors and then determining the aggregate factor rating.

The illustration used in this chapter was kept relatively simple in order to illustrate the method used. Applying the method to a situation with many more SBU business strength factors or many more service area attractiveness factors is not any more difficult, but just involves more work.

Part V

Matrix Analysis Techniques for Mission Departments

The two matrix analysis techniques described above for SBUs can also be applied to the analysis of mission departments of health care organizations. These two techniques are the growth share matrix (GSM) and the service segment analysis-mission department business strength (SSAMDBS) matrix.

In Chapter 13, the growth share matrix is discussed in detail. Its major limitations are that it is based on only two factors—service segment growth rate and relative market share held by mission department—and is therefore largely marketing and market share oriented. An example is provided to illustrate how the matrix analysis technique can be applied.

In Chapter 14, the service segment attractiveness-mission department business strength matrix analysis technique is described in detail. Its major strengths are that it is based on numerous factors from which are extracted through the processes of rating and weighting the two aggregate factors—an aggregate rating of service segment attractiveness and an aggregate rating of mission department business strength.

Chapter 15 uses a hospital case study to illustrate how both the growth share matrix analysis technique and the service segment attractiveness-mission department business strength matrix analysis technique can be applied to a hospital. A comparison of the results of the two matrix analysis techniques is also provided.

Chapter 13

Mission Department Analysis with Growth Share Matrix

13

The growth share matrix in this chapter is used for evaluating mission departments of a health care service organization. Mission departments of health care service organizations deliver such services as inpatient hospitalization, nursing home care, home health care, laboratory services, radiology services, ambulatory health care services, emergency health services, physical and occupational therapy services, etc. as shown on Exhibit 13-1.

GROWTH SHARE MATRIX

The growth share matrix of mission departments is shown in Figure 13-1. The vertical axis measures the annual growth rate of the health care services delivered by the respective mission departments in the service area covered. The horizontal axis measures the relative market share of each mission department in the respective service area. Relative market share is determined by dividing the organization's mission department market share by the market share of the leading competitor. The leading competitor is the mission department with the next highest market share. If the organization's mission department does not have the highest market share, then the leading competitor is the mission department with the highest market share in the service area. In any event the relative market share ratio is always the ratio of the market share of the mission department of the organization being studied to the leading competitor's market share. In the illustration, note that the range of relative market share runs from 0.1 to 1.5, with the dividing line at 0.8. Relative market share figures depend on the mission department of the particular organization, the competitiveness in the service area, and the diversity of the services being provided by the mission department of the organization.

If possible, all services should be plottable within the confines of the selected dimensions. If this is not feasible a mission department can, of

Exhibit 13-1 Examples of Mission Departments in Health Care Organizations

- Inpatient Hospitalization
- Nursing Home Care
- Chemical Laboratory
- Radiology Services
- Ambulatory Medical Services
- Ambulance Service
- Emergency Room Service
- Nursing Home Care
- Occupational Therapy
- Physical Therapy
- Inhalation Therapy
- Surgical Operations
- Renal Dialysis
- Pediatric Services
- Maternity Care

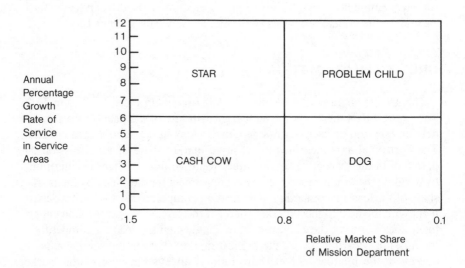

Note: Relative market share is the ratio of the organization's mission department market share to the leading competitor's market share, where the leading competitor is the mission department in the service area with the next highest market share. If the organization's mission department does not have the largest market share, then the leading competitor is the mission department in service area with the largest market share.

Figure 13-1 Growth Share Matrix of Mission Departments

course, always be plotted at the left or right extreme boundary line, which-ever is appropriate. In the same way the annual growth rates of the service segments plotted on the vertical axis are selected so that all mission depart-ments can be plotted on the matrix. In this example, growth rates range from 0 to 12 percent, with the dividing line at 6 percent. If an extremely high or low growth rate needs to be plotted that is off-scale, it can, of course, be located at the upper or lower boundary line.

Both the relative market share and the annual service segment growth rates' dimensions and division lines should be selected so that the various mission departments of the organization can be located across the entire matrix. In other words, the growth share matrix would not reveal very much if all mission departments were located in a single cell, say, the upper right cell of the matrix.

Note that the four cells have been identified by the names of star, cash cow, problem child, and dog. As mentioned before, the appropriateness of the names has been and is still under debate, but their usage is common industry practice. The reader may want to use other names or not use any names at all.

ILLUSTRATION OF THE GROWTH SHARE MATRIX

Suppose that the organization to which the growth share matrix is to be applied is General Hospital. General Hospital has the largest market share, 24 percent, in its service area for the mission department called inpatient hospitalization. It also controls 16 percent of the nursing home market in its service area through three freestanding nursing homes. It recently started a new mission department, a home health care program, but so far has only been able to attain a 3 percent market share in the area it serves. Its mission departments—laboratory and radiology services—control 21 percent and 29 percent of the market, respectively. The mission department of ambulatory care services holds a relatively small market share, 3 percent, because of the proliferation of numerous independent physicians practicing in the area. However, in the emergency health services mission department, General Hospital controls 34 percent of the market through its emergency room. The last mission department, physical and occupational therapy, is combined and covers 13 percent of the market in the service area.

Determining the above market shares for the various mission departments in hospitals within a metropolitan region is not easy. However, it is often surprising how much the directors of your mission departments know about what is going on in their competitors' mission departments of the same specialization. Hence, although exact figures are difficult to obtain, appropri-ate estimates can be made.

The growth rate of each of the services provided by the mission departments varies. The service segment, inpatient hospitalization, has a 1 percent annual growth rate; the service segment, nursing home care, is growing at a 7 percent annual rate; the service segment, home health care, is the most rapidly growing service at 11 percent annually; the service segments, laboratory and radiological services, are each growing at a 4 percent growth rate; the service segments, ambulatory health care and emergency care services, are each growing at 5 percent annual rates; and the service segment, physical and occupational therapy services, is growing at a 10 percent annual rate.

General Hospital is the market share leader in inpatient hospitalization, nursing homes, radiology services, and emergency care services. In the other areas General Hospital has strengths, but is not a leader. The next major competitor in inpatient hospitalization has a 15 percent market share, in nursing home care the next major competitor has a 10 percent market share, in radiology services the next major market share leader has 10 percent, and in emergency health care services the next leading competitor has 14 percent. In service segments where General Hospital does not have the leading market share, the market share leaders have market shares of 20 percent in home health care, of 25 percent in laboratory services, of 6 percent in ambulatory health care services, and of 18 percent in physical and occupational therapy services. These market shares and percentage growth rates for the services and respective mission departments are shown in Table 13-1.

Table 13-1 Summary of Service Segment's Growth Rates, Mission Department's Market Shares and Leading Competitor Market Shares: General Hospital

Service/Mission Department	Service Segment Growth Rate	Mission Department Market Share	Leading Competitor Market Share	Relative Market Share*
Inpatient hospitalization (IHC)	1	24	15	1.6
Nursing home care (NHC)	7	16	10	1.6
Home health care (HHC)	11	3	20	0.15
Laboratory services (LS)	4	21	25	0.84
Radiology services (RS)	4	29	10	2.90
Ambulatory health services (AHS)	5	3	6	0.50
Emergency health services (EHS)	5	34	14	2.43
Physical and occupational therapy services (POTS)	10	13	18	0.72

* Relative market share is the ratio of General Hospital's mission department's market share to its leading competitor's market share.

Based on the summarized data, each mission department can now be plotted on the growth share matrix as shown in Figure 13-2. Note that the relative market share scale on the horizontal axis ranges from 0 to 3.0 to satisfy the range of relative market shares of the eight mission departments. The annual percentage growth rate ranges from 0 to 12 percent. Only one mission department, nursing home care, falls in the star category. The mission departments, laboratory services and ambulatory health services, are classified as dogs; the mission departments, home health care and physical and occupational therapy services, are problem children; and the remaining three mission departments—radiology services, emergency health services, and inpatient hospitalization services—fall in the cash cow category.

Whether the assigned categories are correct is, of course, up for debate. Remember that the growth share matrix only considers relative market share of the mission department and service segment growth rate. There is no

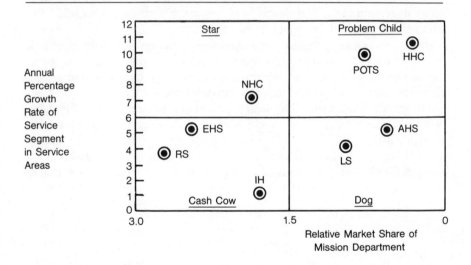

Note: Relative market share is the ratio of the mission department's market share to its leading competitor's market share.

RS-radiology services
EHS-emergency health care services
IH-inpatient hospitalization
NHC-nursing home care
POTS-physical and occupational therapy services
HHC-home health care services
LS-laboratory services
AHS-ambulatory health care services

Figure 13-2 Growth Share Matrix of General Hospital

consideration of profitability and potential market share growth rate. For instance, given General Hospital's domination in several health care service segments in the service area, it seems likely that continued aggressive marketing should enable it to increase considerably its market share of home health services. As a result the mission department, home health services, could quickly move from a problem child designation to a star designation.

The above information can be used by a hospital's planning group to determine priorities and goals for the future. It also indicates how good or effective a hospital's mission departments are in relation to their competitors' mission departments.

SUMMARY

In this chapter the growth share matrix was applied to a hospital with eight mission departments. The matrix was constructed so that it satisfied the parameters of each of the eight mission departments.

It is important to recognize the limitations of the growth share matrix. It only measures relative market share and the service segment's growth rate in the service area. Hence, no information is collected on profitability, cash flows, or compatibility with other mission departments.

The growth share matrix has been popular over the years and still remains popular because it is relatively easy to apply, it requires data that are widely available and produces results that are, at least at first glance, easy to understand. Chapter 14 discusses an alternative to the growth share matrix that is more difficult and time consuming to apply, but produces more usable results.

Mission Department Evaluation with Service Segment Attractiveness-Mission Department Business Strength Matrix

HIGHLIGHTS

- Service Segment Attractiveness-Mission Department Business Strength Matrix
- Illustration of the Service Segment Attractiveness-Mission Department Business Strength Matrix
- Summary

184

14

The service segment attractiveness—mission department business strength (SSAMDBS) matrix is generally attributed to the General Electric Corporation, which presumably used it because of the limitations of the growth share matrix. Both the growth share matrix and the SSAMDBS matrix were developed to evaluate SBUs of larger corporations. The SSAMDBS matrix can also be used to evaluate mission departments of a health care service organization.

SERVICE SEGMENT ATTRACTIVENESS-MISSION DEPARTMENT BUSINESS STRENGTH MATRIX

The framework of a typical service segment attractiveness-mission department business strength matrix (SSAMDBS) is shown in Figure 14-1. The vertical axis measures the mission department's business strength in serving the respective service segment, and the horizontal axis measures the attractiveness of the respective service segment. Note that the axes are measured on a 2.0 to 3.5 scale. This scale is used because the various factors that determine the mission department business strength and the service segment attractiveness are measured on a 1 to 4 scale, where the scale ranges from poor (1) to strong (4) for business strength and from unattractive (1) to attractive (4) for the service segment's service area attractiveness. Because almost any factor will at least receive some positive evaluation the actual range of the aggregated factors falls commonly between 2.0 and 3.5.

Examples of mission department business strength factors are financial, marketing, quality of services, accessibility, and others as shown in Exhibit 14-1. Exhibit 14-2 shows examples of service segment attractiveness, including growth rate, profitability, ease of entry, and competitiveness. Each one of the factors is assigned a rating between 1 and 4, and each is weighted. The

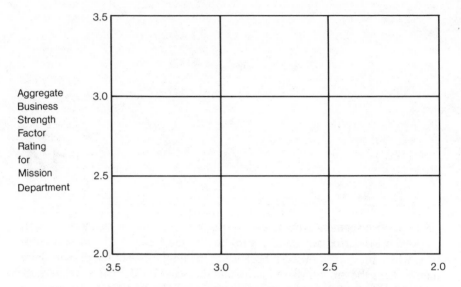

Aggregate Attractiveness Factor Rating for Service Segment

Figure 14-1 A Typical Service Segment Attractiveness-Mission Department Business Strength Matrix: Service Segment Evaluation

---

Exhibit 14-1 Examples of Mission Department Business Strength Factors

- Financial
- Marketing
- Quality of Services
- Facility Location
- Employee Turnover
- Reputation
- Market Share
- Service Comprehensiveness
- Price Competitiveness
- Promotion Effectiveness
- Productivity
- Quality of Staff
- General Image

Exhibit 14-2 Examples of Service Segment Attractiveness Factors

- Annual Growth Rate
- Profitability
- Ease of Entry
- Competitiveness
- Salary Levels
- Physician Supply
- Allied Personnel Supply
- Regulation
- Taxation
- Local Government Support

weighted ratings are then aggregated into an overall measure of mission department business strength and service segment attractiveness.

Table 14-1 shows how ratings and weights are aggregated for the mission department business strength component. The aggregation of service segment attractiveness factors for a service segment is shown in Table 14-2. The figures are arbitrary and are chosen only for purposes of illustration. Note that in all cases the weights applied to the factors must add up to 1.00 in order to obtain an unbiased aggregate measure.

In the case of the service segment attractiveness factors, ease of entry is given a low value of 1 if it is easy to enter that particular service segment for a new organization, and conversely, a high value of 4 is assigned if it is very difficult to enter that particular service segment. If ease of entry is high, then more competitors are bound to enter the market and thus make the service segment less attractive. Competitiveness is given a low value of 1 if there is strong competition and a high value of 4 if competition is weak. Weak competition enhances the attractiveness of the service segment.

Table 14-1 Aggregation of Mission Department Business Strength Factor Ratings: Service Segment Evaluation

Mission Department Business Strength Factors	Rating	Weight	Rating × Weight
Financial	2.0	0.25	0.50
Marketing	1.5	0.40	0.60
Quality of services	3.0	0.25	0.75
Accessibility	2.5	0.10	0.25
Aggregate rating		1.00	2.10

Table 14-2 Aggregation of Service Segment Attractiveness Factor Ratings: Service Segment Evaluation

Service Segment Attractiveness Factors	Rating	Weight	Rating × Weight
Growth rate	1.5	0.40	0.60
Profitability	2.0	0.20	0.40
Ease of entry	1.8	0.30	0.54
Competitiveness	2.1	0.10	0.21
Aggregate rating		1.00	1.75

ILLUSTRATION OF THE SSAMDBS MATRIX

The organization to which the SSAMDBS matrix is applied here is General Hospital, the same hospital discussed in Chapter 13. General Hospital is active in eight service segments and wants to evaluate each of the mission departments serving those segments using the SSAMDBS matrix. The eight mission departments are inpatient hospitalization, nursing home care, home health care, laboratory services, radiology services, ambulatory health services, emergency health services, and physical and occupational therapy services.

Senior and operating management developed for each of the eight mission departments aggregate service segment attractiveness factor ratings and aggregate mission department business strength factor ratings. The service segment attractiveness factors that senior and operating management identified were the same for all eight service segments; they were service segment growth rate, profitability of service segment, ease of entry for service segment, competitiveness of service segment, and regulation effects of service segments.

For each of the eight mission departments the aggregate service segment attractiveness factor rating was determined as illustrated for one mission department, nursing home care, in Table 14-3. Note that excessive regulation usually adversely affects the attractiveness of a service segment, at least in

Table 14-3 Aggregation of Service Segment Attractiveness Factor Ratings for Nursing Home Care

Service Segment Attractiveness Factors	Rating	Weight	Rating × Weight
Service segment growth rate	3.0	.25	.75
Profitability	2.0	.30	.60
Ease of entry	3.0	.10	.30
Competitiveness	2.5	.10	.25
Regulation effects	1.5	.25	.38
Aggregate rating		1.00	2.28

the health care sector. As a result the rating of 1.5 for regulation effects indicates a low attractiveness of the service segment.

This procedure to determine the service segment attractiveness factor rating is repeated for each of the other seven mission departments.

The next step is to determine the aggregate mission department business strength factor ratings for each of the eight mission departments. Senior management identified five business strength factors that it wants to use to determine the aggregate business strength factor rating for each of the eight mission departments. The five business strength factors are financial, marketing, quality of service, accessibility and staff competence.

Table 14-4 illustrates how senior management determined the aggregate business strength factor rating for the mission department home health care services. Note that one of General Hospital's particular business strengths was accessibility because the hospital was located in the center of a relatively older population whose need for home health care was quite great. The other business strengths were quality of services and staff competence. General Hospital's extensive experience and good reputation in patient care enabled it to attract high-quality personnel, which, in turn, contributed a good deal to these two business strengths.

The above procedure to determine the aggregate mission department business strength factor rating for home health care services was repeated for the other seven mission departments. The results are shown in Table 14-5 and include both the aggregate mission department business strength factor ratings and the aggregate service segment attractiveness factor ratings for all eight mission departments.

The next step in the mission department analysis evaluation using the SSAMDBS matrix approach is to plot each of the eight mission departments on the SSAMDBS matrix. This has been done and is shown on Figure 14-2. In both the growth share matrix and the SSAMDBS matrix, the most desirable mission department appears in the upper left corner of the matrix. Conversely, the least desirable mission departments appear in the lower right corner. Note that the mission department with the highest aggregate factor

Table 14-4 Aggregation of Mission Department Business Strength Factor Ratings for Home Health Care

Mission Department Business Strength Factors	Rating	Weight	Rating × Weight
Financial	2.5	.10	.25
Marketing	1.5	.30	.45
Quality of services	3.0	.25	.75
Accessibility	3.0	.10	.30
Staff competence	3.6	.25	.90
Aggregate rating		1.00	2.65

Table 14-5 Aggregate Factor Ratings for Service Segment Attractiveness and Mission Department Business Strength

Mission Departments	Aggregate Service Segment Attractiveness Factor Ratings	Aggregate Mission Department Business Strength Factor Ratings
Inpatient hospitalization (IH)	2.40	3.16
Nursing home care (NHC)	2.28	3.06
Home health care (HHC)	3.34	2.65
Laboratory services (LS)	2.68	2.38
Radiology services (RS)	3.09	2.42
Ambulatory health services (AHS)	2.21	2.65
Emergency health services (EHS)	3.09	3.16
Physical and occupational therapy services (POTS)	2.80	2.90

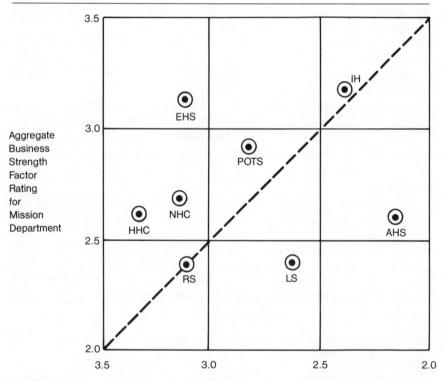

Aggregate Service Segment Attractiveness Factor Rating

Figure 14-2 Service Segment Attractiveness-Mission Department Business Strength Matrix: General Hospital

ratings for both mission department business strength and service segment attractiveness is emergency health services (EHS). In this case not a single mission department fell in the lower right corner of the SSAMDBS matrix.

In general, mission departments falling in the upper left triangle of the SSAMDBS matrix are quite attractive and usually have a promising future as profit and growth contributors to the organization. Mission departments segments falling in the lower right triangle of the SSAMDBS matrix are usually potential problems. In some cases they may be resuscitated by management action. However, especially if the aggregate service segment attractiveness factor rating is low, senior management may not have much influence on improving the overall SSAMDBS matrix status of the mission department.

In this example, General Hospital's mission departments are doing quite well. Only two mission departments are in the lower right triangle of the SSAMDBS matrix, two are close to the borderline separating the two triangles, and four mission departments are clearly located in the upper left triangle of the SSAMDBS matrix.

SUMMARY

In this chapter the service segment attractiveness-mission department business strength matrix was applied to a hospital with eight mission departments. The SSAMDBS matrix was constructed so that it fit the parameters of each of the eight mission departments.

Although the SSAMDBS approach has limitations its evaluation of mission departments is much more comprehensive than the growth share matrix discussed in Chapter 13. Whereas the growth share matrix largely measures mission department market share and service segment growth rate, the SSAMDBS matrix also measures several dimensions of mission department business strength and service segment attractiveness. Mission department business strength is measured in terms of financial, marketing, staff competence, accessibility, and quality of services delivered. Service segment attractiveness is measured in terms of growth rate, profitability, ease of entry, competitiveness, and regulation effects.

The disadvantage of the SSAMDBS matrix, in comparison with the growth share matrix, is the added work involved in evaluating the various factors that determine mission department business strength and service segment attractiveness. However, the work involved in evaluating all factors will provide senior management with a deeper and more extensive knowledge of the factors that determine whether a mission department is a poor or good performer. The extensive evaluation and analysis also determine whether a mission department should receive particular attention and resources because of the promise it shows in the strategic plan of the organization.

Case Illustration of the Growth Share Matrix and the Service Segment Attractiveness-Mission Department Business Strength Matrix

This chapter shows how the growth share matrix and the service segment attractiveness-mission department business strength (SSAMDBS) matrix can be applied to a case study of a typical general hospital, to which is assigned the name Kenmore Hospital. The application of the two matrices reveals the limitations of the growth share matrix and points out clearly the need for the more detailed factor evaluation approach embodied in the SSAMDBS matrix.

CASE A: ANALYSIS AND EVALUATION OF MISSION DEPARTMENTS USING THE GROWTH SHARE MATRIX

Kenmore Hospital is one of seven hospitals in a Midwestern city with a population of about 450,000 people. The hospital provides a comprehensive array of health care services, including intensive care, renal dialysis, and 13 other services provided by a total of 15 mission departments.

Mr. Alan Brown, the vice president of planning, had asked the accounting department to prepare a listing of the revenues and direct expenses associated with each of the 15 mission departments (Table 15-1). The largest mission department by far was medical and surgical inpatient services, which provided over one-third of all hospital revenues.

To aid in the evaluating of the 15 mission departments, Mr. Brown decided to develop and use the growth share matrix (GSM). Information was therefore required on the market shares of every mission department of Kenmore Hospital and of their respective leading competitors, as well as annual growth rates for each service segment served by each mission department. Mr. Brown collected the necessary information from the state health department planning staff and from hospital utilization reports. Collecting market share data is a very time-consuming process. In most states, business strength and

Table 15-1 Kenmore Hospital: Revenues and Expenses for Year Ending
December 31, 1986

Mission Department/Service Segment	Revenues	Expenses
Medical and surgical inpatient services	$1,037,225	$ 545,874
OB-GYN, delivery room, and nursery	116,135	93,449
Intensive care unit	65,000	51,262
Surgical operations	159,650	93,554
Miscellaneous services	211,698	102,567
Renal dialysis	19,500	7,778
Emergency room	88,780	74,071
Laboratory	308,206	216,564
EKG	40,080	29,243
X-ray and nuclear medicine	238,431	124,305
Pharmacy	346,836	169,551
Anesthesiology	89,800	62,749
Respiratory therapy	142,738	42,434
Physical and occupational therapy	27,095	21,844
Ambulance services	68,325	108,873
Total	$2,959,499	$1,744,118

service segment attractiveness data for mission departments are not available. Sample studies are often used instead.

The data are summarized on Table 15-2. Note that the mission department with the largest market share, 30 percent, is respiratory therapy. The smallest market share is 8 percent, which is held by the hospital's ambulance services. The annual service segment growth rates range from 2 percent for surgical operations to 6 percent for physical and occupational therapy. Mr. Brown reviewed the collected data on the 15 mission departments and began developing the Growth Share Matrix.

CASE B: ANALYSIS AND EVALUATION OF MISSION DEPARTMENTS USING THE SERVICE SEGMENT ATTRACTIVENESS-MISSION DEPARTMENT BUSINESS STRENGTH MATRIX

To aid in the evaluation of 15 mission departments, Mr. Alan Brown, vice president of planning, decided to use the service segment attractiveness-mission department business strength (SSAMDBS) matrix. For the SSAMDBS matrix to be applied information was required on the various factors that determine the service segment attractiveness of each service segment and the business strength of each service segment mission department.

Table 15-2 Distribution of Market Shares and Service Segment Growth Rates in Areas Served by Kenmore Hospital

Mission Department/ Service Segment	Kenmore Market Share %	Leading Competitor Market Share %	Annual Service Segment Growth Rate %
Medical and surgical inpatient services	20	22	3
OB-GYN, delivery room, and nursery	24	18	3
Intensive care unit	18	20	4
Surgical operations	19	17	2
Miscellaneous services	26	21	5
Renal dialysis	10	32	4
Emergency room	23	20	3
Laboratories	16	20	5
EKG	19	15	4
X-ray and nuclear medicine	32	16	5
Pharmacy	23	15	4
Anesthesiology	20	18	3
Respiratory therapy	30	12	5
Physical and occupational therapy	12	20	6
Ambulance services	8	19	4

Note: The leading competitor is the market share leader in the respective service segment, unless Kenmore is the leader. Then, the leading competitor has the second highest market share.

Table 15-3 shows the business strength factor ratings for each of the 15 mission departments. The four mission department business strength factors are marketing, quality of services, accessibility, and competence of staff. In addition a weight for each of the four factors was developed by Kenmore Hospital's management group and is shown at the bottom of the table. The weight of the four mission department business strength factors ranges from .10 to .40.

The service segment attractiveness factor ratings for the 15 service segments are shown on Table 15-4. The five service segment attractiveness factors are service segment growth rate, profitability, ease of entry, competitiveness, and regulation effects. At the bottom of the table are listed the weights of the factors. The weights range from .10 to .35 and were determined by Mr. Brown in consultation with Kenmore Hospital's senior management group.

Mr. Brown reviewed the collected data on the 15 mission departments segments and began the calculations required to apply the service segment attractiveness-mission department business strength matrix.

Table 15-3 Business Strength Factor Ratings of Kenmore Hospital Mission Departments (Scale:1–4)

Mission Department/ Service Segment	Marketing	Quality of Services	Accessibility	Competence of Staff
Medical and surgical inpatient services	3.0	3.5	3.0	3.0
OB-GYN, delivery room, and nursery	2.5	3.5	3.0	4.0
Intensive care unit	3.5	4.0	3.0	3.5
Surgical operations	3.5	3.5	3.0	3.5
Miscellaneous services	2.5	3.0	3.0	3.0
Renal dialysis	2.5	2.0	3.0	2.5
Emergency room	3.0	4.0	3.5	3.5
Laboratories	3.0	3.0	2.5	3.0
EKG	2.5	3.0	2.5	3.5
X-ray and nuclear medicine	3.0	3.5	3.0	3.5
Pharmacy	2.0	3.5	2.5	3.0
Anesthesiology	3.0	4.0	3.5	3.5
Respiratory therapy	2.5	3.0	2.5	3.5
Physical and occupational therapy	2.0	3.0	2.5	3.0
Ambulance services	2.0	2.5	2.0	2.0
Weighting of factors	.20	.30	.10	.40

ANALYSIS AND EVALUATION OF CASE A AND CASE B BY THE TWO MATRIX SYSTEMS

Analysis of Kenmore Hospital with the growth share matrix (GSM) and the service segment attractiveness-mission department business strength (SSAMDBS) matrix shows the mechanics of using each approach and the difference in the depth of information they provide. GSM uses relative market share of mission department and service segment growth rate on a two-by-two matrix. Development of the SSAMDBS matrix is a more complex process, but it yields detailed information that provides a stronger foundation for strategic planning. The two dimensions of this matrix, service segment attractiveness and mission department business strength, are aggregates of factor ratings determined by management.

Growth Share Matrix

Kenmore Hospital's services are provided through 15 mission departments; Kenmore Hospital is the leading competitor, in terms of market share, in 9 of the 15 service segments as shown in Table 15-5. Relative market shares of mission departments and annual service segment growth rates are plotted on the vertical and horizontal axes of the growth share matrix as shown on

Table 15-4 Service Segment Attractiveness Factor Ratings of Kenmore Hospital Mission Departments (Scale:1–4)

Mission Department/ Service Segment	Service Segment Growth Rate	Profitibility	Ease of Entry	Competitiveness	Regulation Effects
Medical and surgical inpatient services	2.0	3.5	4.0	2.5	3.5
OB-GYN, delivery room, and nursery	2.0	2.8	4.0	2.5	3.0
Intensive care unit	2.7	2.8	4.0	2.5	3.5
Surgical operations	1.3	3.2	4.0	2.5	3.5
Miscellaneous services	3.3	3.5	2.5	1.5	2.5
Renal dialysis	2.7	3.7	2.0	1.5	3.0
Emergency room	2.0	2.7	3.5	3.0	3.5
Laboratories	3.3	3.1	1.5	2.0	3.0
EKG	2.7	3.0	1.0	2.0	3.0
X-ray and nuclear medicine	3.3	3.5	1.5	3.0	3.0
Pharmacy	2.7	3.5	2.0	3.0	3.0
Anesthesiology	2.0	3.1	4.0	4.0	3.5
Respiratory therapy	3.3	4.0	2.0	2.5	3.0
Physical and occupational therapy	4.0	2.8	1.5	1.5	2.0
Ambulance services	2.7	1.0	1.0	1.5	2.0
Weighting of factors	.20	.35	.15	.20	.10

Figure 15-1. The labels in each of the four cells reflect the traditional designations of star, cash cow, problem child, and dog for the mission departments that fall within each cell.

The mission departments that are identified as stars are respiratory therapy, x-ray and nuclear medicine, and pharmacy. All three have strong relative market shares and high annual growth rates. The mission departments identified as dogs are OB-GYN, delivery room, and nursery; emergency room; medical and surgical inpatient services; anesthesiology, and surgical operations. They are all weak in terms of relative market share and service segment annual growth rates. The remaining mission departments are identified as problem children. They have high annual service segment growth rates but a weak relative market share. The growth share matrix does not provide enough information to assess the potential growth of these problematic mission departments if marketing efforts are improved. Nor does it indicate whether profitability is sufficient to warrant the expense of an improved marketing effort. It leaves these questions to management's judgment. The SSAMDBS matrix, although it requires more data from management, also provides better insight into the hospital's position.

Table 15-5 Distribution of Market Share and Service Segment Growth Rates for Mission Departments of Kenmore Hospital

Service Segment/ Mission Department	Kenmore Market Share %	Leading Competitor Market Share %	Kenmore Relative Market Share %	Annual Service Segment Growth Rate %
Medical and surgical inpatient services	20	22	0.91	3
OB-GYN, delivery room, and nursery	24	18	1.33	3
Intensive care unit	18	20	0.90	4
Surgical operations	19	17	1.12	2
Miscellaneous services	26	21	1.24	5
Renal dialysis	10	32	0.31	4
Emergency room	23	20	1.15	3
Laboratories	16	20	0.80	5
X-ray and nuclear medicine	32	16	2.00	5
Pharmacy	23	15	1.53	4
Anesthesiology	20	18	1.11	3
Respiratory therapy	30	12	2.50	5
Physical and occupational therapy	12	20	0.60	6
Ambulance services	8	18	0.44	4

Service Segment Attractiveness-Mission Department Business Strength Matrix

The SSAMDBS requires the identification of two sets of factor ratings. One set of factor ratings reflects the attractiveness of the service segment in general, and another set measures the specific mission department's business strength in that service area. The factors for both the mission department's business strength and the service segment's attractiveness are given weights, and an aggregate rating is calculated. The aggregate ratings for each mission department are then plotted on the three-by-three SSAMDBS matrix.

Kenmore Hospital's management has selected five factors of service segment attractiveness: growth rate, profitability, ease of entry, competitiveness, and regulation effects. Management assigned a rating to each factor on a 1 to 4 scale, with 4 indicating the most attractive and 1 indicating the least attractive. Too, management identified four factors of mission department business strength: marketing, quality of service, accessibility, and staff competence. Each factor was then assigned a rating on a 1 to 4 scale, with 4 indicating high business strength and 1 indicating low business strength.

Each of the five factors for service segment attractiveness was then assigned a relative weight so that the sum of the weights added up to 1.00.

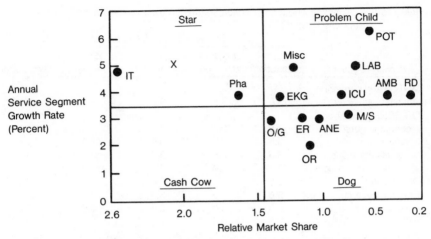

Legend:

M/S = Medical and surgical inpatient services
O/G = OB/GYN, delivery room, and nursery
ICU = Intensive care unit
OR = Operating room
Misc = Miscellaneous
RD = Renal dialysis
ER = Emergency room
LAB = Laboratories
EKG = EKG
X = X-ray and nuclear medicine
Pha = Pharmacy
ANE = Anesthesiology
IT = Respiratory therapy
POT = Physical and occupational therapy
AMB = Ambulance services

Figure 15-1 Growth Share Matrix for Kenmore Hospital

Similarly, each of the four mission department business strength factors were assigned a relative weight such that the sum of the weights equaled one.

For each mission department, aggregate ratings for service segment attractiveness and mission department business strength were calculated, based on the respective factor ratings and weights as shown on Table 15-6. The aggregate ratings were then plotted on a SSAMDBS matrix to obtain a composite view of the relative service segment attractiveness and business strengths of the 15 mission departments (Figure 15-2).

As is true for the growth share matrix, the mission departments with the best potential are in the upper left corner and the mission departments with the worst potential are in the lower right corner. However, unlike the growth

Table 15-6 Business Strength and Service Segment Attractiveness Factor Ratings for Kenmore Hospital

Service Segement	Business Strength Factor Ratings				
	Marketing	Quality of Services	Accessibility	Staff Competence	Aggregate
Medical and surgical inpatient services	3.0	3.5	3.0	3.0	3.2
OB-GYN, delivery room, and nursery	2.5	3.5	3.0	4.0	3.5
Intensive care unit	3.5	4.0	3.0	3.5	3.6
Surgical operations	3.5	3.5	3.0	3.5	3.5
Miscellaneous services	2.5	3.0	3.0	3.0	2.9
Renal dialysis	2.5	2.0	3.0	2.5	2.4
Emergency room	3.0	4.0	3.5	3.5	3.6
Laboratories	3.0	3.0	2.5	3.0	3.0
EKG	2.5	3.0	2.5	3.5	3.1
X-ray and nuclear medicine	3.0	3.5	3.0	3.5	3.4
Pharmacy	2.0	3.5	2.5	3.0	2.9
Anesthesiology	3.0	4.0	3.5	3.5	3.6
Respiratory therapy	2.5	3.0	2.5	3.5	3.1
Physical and occupational therapy	2.0	3.0	2.5	3.0	2.8
Ambulance services	2.0	2.5	2.0	2.0	2.2
Weighting of factors	.20	.30	.10	.40	

share matrix, the SSAMDBS matrix allows management to review the preliminary data, shown in Table 15-6, to consider the strengths and weaknesses of mission departments with medium/high aggregate ratings and those with medium/low aggregate ratings.

Close to the diagonal, on and above it, are the mission departments with medium/high aggregate ratings. They are EKG, laboratories, miscellaneous services, and pharmacy. The first three mission departments have good business strength but poor service segment attractiveness, largely because they are easy to enter and thus quite competitive. Pharmacy's attractiveness received a higher aggregate rating than its business strength. For all four mission departments, weakness of the business strength factors results from poor marketing efforts and/or poor access locations. It appears that each of these mission departments is maintained as a support service to the major functions of the hospital and that management is not interested in developing them further. Yet, increased marketing efforts and establishment of more accessible satellite operations for the laboratories, miscellaneous services, and pharmacy might make these necessary mission departments stronger profit generators. The low service segment attractiveness score of EKG suggests that it is unlikely to grow.

Service Segment Attractiveness
Factor Ratings

Svce. Seg. Growth Rate	Profitability	Ease of Entry	Competitiveness	Regulation Effects	Aggregate
2.0	3.5	4.0	2.5	3.5	3.1
2.0	2.8	4.0	2.5	3.0	2.8
2.7	2.8	4.0	2.5	3.5	3.0
1.3	3.2	4.0	2.5	3.5	2.8
3.3	3.5	2.5	1.5	2.5	2.8
2.7	3.7	2.0	1.5	3.0	2.7
2.0	2.7	3.5	3.0	3.5	2.8
3.3	3.1	1.5	2.0	3.0	2.7
2.7	3.0	1.0	2.0	3.0	2.4
3.3	3.5	1.5	3.0	3.0	3.0
2.7	3.5	2.0	3.0	3.0	3.0
2.0	3.1	4.0	4.0	3.5	3.2
3.3	4.0	2.0	2.5	3.0	3.2
4.0	2.8	1.5	1.5	2.0	2.5
2.7	1.0	1.0	1.5	2.0	1.5
.20	.35	.15	.20	.10	

Two other mission departments, physical and occupational therapy (POT) and renal dialysis (RD), have weak aggregate ratings in both dimensions and should be considered either for future strengthening or reduction. POT has the advantage of having high quality service and competent staff, both of which contribute to its business strength. However, marketing is weak and detracts from its business strength. POT's attractiveness is bolstered by exceptional growth, but profitability is only modest and ease of entry, competition, and regulation all are rated low. Renal dialysis lacks quality service and staff competence; its marketing is also weak. As has POT, it has easy entry and strong competition, but its profitability, not growth, is particularly strong. Given the impressive strength of Kenmore Hospital's core mission departments, Kenmore should consider efforts to develop one or both of these areas. Development of physical and occupational therapy should be less extensive because it already has good quality service and competent staff. However, both of these factors should be improved for renal dialysis if Kenmore is going to provide this service at all. Otherwise, renal dialysis detracts from the high standards that Kenmore Hospital maintains.

Strict interpretation of Kenmore Hospital's SSAMDBS matrix could yield a definite strategic plan as shown in Figure 15-3. However, judgment plays a

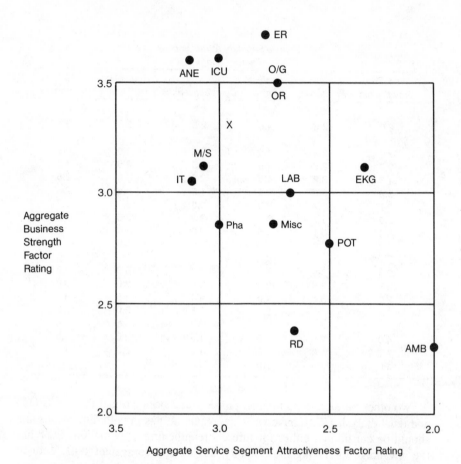

Figure 15-2 Service Segment Attractiveness-Business Strength Matrix for Kenmore Hospital

vital role in the matrix evaluation system also, and it should be treated as the important tool that it is. A hospital may need to provide a loss-generator, such as ambulance services, to maintain disaster preparedness and to maintain community goodwill. Furthermore, in spite of the abundance of information that the SSAMDBS considers, there are always other factors that occur to an astute management team.

The information provided by the two matrix systems is not just different in detail but also in direction. For six mission departments—medical and surgical inpatient services; OB-GYN, delivery room, and nursery; intensive care unit, surgical operations, emergency room, and anesthesiology—the matrices yield diametrically opposed results. These differences are caused by the simplistic two-dimensional approach of the growth share matrix that fails to

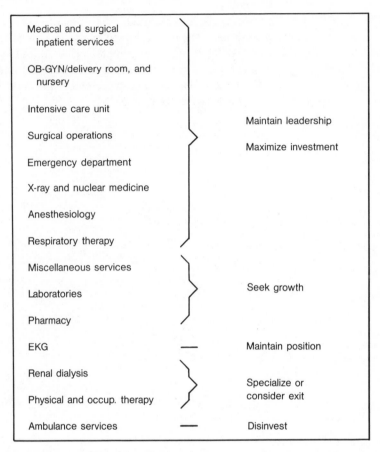

Figure 15-3 Strategy for Kenmore Hospital Based on Strict Interpretation of the SSAMDBS

consider many important factors, particularly the exceptional quality of Kenmore's core mission departments and the strong profitability and barriers to entry of these service segments.

SUMMARY

The growth share matrix and the SSAMDBS matrix are useful tools for studying a hospital's mission departments in terms of their relative business strength and the attractiveness of each service segment. The essential difference between the two matrices is in the complexity of the mission department business strength and the service segment attractiveness ratings. For the growth share matrix, only two dimensions are used, relative market share and service segment annual growth rate. The measure used by the SSAMDBS are aggregates of multiple factors. The increased complexity of compiling a SSAMDBS matrix yields a reward of greater depth of information. But the user must still be alert for factors that are not represented and also for mistaken, perhaps biased, estimates of factor ratings.

Part VI

Strategic Management in Nonhospital Health Care Organizations

Although the hospital is still by far the most dominant health care institution, other health care institutions are rapidly emerging and are becoming separate industries within the overall health care industry. The three health care institutions addressed in this section are ambulatory health care centers, health maintenance organizations (HMOs), and home health care organizations.

Chapter 16 covers strategic management issues in ambulatory health care centers. Specifically addressed is the strategy of vertical integration by which hospitals acquire or develop ambulatory care centers and urgent care centers in order to gain a captive market for hospital admissions and procedures.

Chapter 17 discusses in detail the strategic planning development problems associated with developing new HMOs. The HMO may be likely to be vertically integrated into the hospital because of the logical connection between ambulatory care, the HMO's specialty, and inpatient care, the hospital's specialty. Not many hospitals have the expertise to plan and develop HMOs, but those same hospitals are certainly in a position to merge with or capture existing HMOs.

Chapter 18, the last chapter in this part, addresses strategic management issues related to home health care organizations. Four types of home health care organizations are identified. Again the hospital seems to be in a perfect position to integrate vertically by either acquiring or developing home health care organizations.

Chapter 16

Strategic Management for Ambulatory Health Care Centers

- Different Types of Ambulatory Health Care Centers
- Supply and Demand of Physicians
- Demand for Convenience Ambulatory Care
- Strategic Planning for Ambulatory Care Centers
- Summary

16

This chapter addresses the issue of strategic planning for ambulatory health care facilities. Ambulatory health care facilities are those facilities organized to deliver comprehensive outpatient care on an appointment or walk-in basis. Comprehensive outpatient care generally includes basic family, outpatient emergency, pediatric, obstretrics and gynecology, and other types of health care that can be delivered on an outpatient basis.

Haley, in a 1984 article, noted that ambulatory care was undergoing and will continue to undergo a period of restructuring in response to a number of environmental forces.[1] The most important environmental force is the increase in competitiveness of the medical profession because of a surplus of physicians in certain specialties. Another force is the reduction in the demand for inpatient hospital care because of the prospective payment movement initiated by the Medicare diagnostic-related groupings (DRGs). This movement also has led to a significant increase in competitiveness among hospitals. The third force is the demand for ambulatory care that is more convenient in terms of location—close to patients' homes—and time—evening and weekends as opposed to daylight hours on a Monday-to-Friday basis. This chapter considers the restructuring of ambulatory health care.

DIFFERENT TYPES OF AMBULATORY HEALTH CARE CENTERS

There are a wide variety of ambulatory health care facilities. The most common, of course, is the physician's office, especially the solo practitioner's office. Its services are usually limited to the specialty of the physician. The solo physician's office will be probably supplanted during the next 20 years by the newer types of ambulatory health care centers discussed below.

Such offices will most likely be merged into larger, multiphysician facilities that will either provide multispecialty or highly specialized care.

The next most common ambulatory care center is the group practice office from which a group of physicians practice. It is usually considerably more elaborate than the solo practitioner's office and may employ large support staff of nurses, laboratory technicians, x-ray technicians, office staff, and an office manager. It may cover a variety of specialties, such as basic primary care and some of the more common specialties. It may also be centered around one specialty, such as family practice, OB-GYN, pediatrics, or orthopedics.

A newer type of ambulatory care center is one that provides what is often called convenience medicine. Such a center may be called an urgent care center or, if local and state law allows, an emergency care center. It is typically located in convenient locations with heavy population traffic, such as shopping centers. It is usually open evenings, weekends, and holidays when most other ambulatory care centers are closed. An urgent care center is typically staffed by at least one physician and several support personnel, such as receptionists, nurses, and technicians. To ensure that the cost per visit is kept low, overhead costs are carefully controlled. To encourage utilization, extensive use of advertising is made, often to the dismay of the established medical profession. In many respects it provides an alternative to the much higher cost of hospital emergency room care.

The above three types of ambulatory care centers represent the vast majority of the ambulatory care market, except for those facilities located in hospitals. Hospital ambulatory care centers are the emergency room for emergency care of any level of severity, and the hospital outpatient clinics, which are more commonly found in university hospitals or those in medically underserved areas. These outpatient clinics are quite similar to urgent care centers in that they often provide walk-in care, as well as scheduled medical care. Outpatient clinics may provide both primary and specialty care. They are often staffed by medical residents.

Another type of ambulatory care center is the ambulatory surgical center where "same day" surgery is performed. Patients walk in on their own and also leave on the same day. There are both freestanding and hospital-based ambulatory surgery centers. Finally, mental health clinics provide mental health counseling on an appointment basis and can be freestanding or hospital-based.

Most ambulatory care facilities have affiliations with local hospitals, largely through physician staff privileges with those hospitals. Although only a limited number of freestanding ambulatory care centers are currently owned by hospitals, in the future many more will be wholly or partially owned by them because of the stronger ties that hospitals will want with the ambulatory care market. These ties are necessary to ensure that hospitals will have a steady supply of referred patients to fill their beds and use their referral services. Acquiring freestanding ambulatory care centers is a form of rearward vertical integration or distribution channel enhancement.

SUPPLY AND DEMAND OF PHYSICIANS

The supply and demand of physicians is an important factor in determining the pace at which the ambulatory care sector will be restructured. There had been a shortage of physicians in nearly all specialties until the early 1980s. Because of this shortage, development of multiphysician ambulatory care centers controlled and owned by nonphysicians was slow. In addition, physician income levels were relatively quite high, and salaries to attract physicians to work for ambulatory care centers were similarly high. Because physicians form a major part of ambulatory care center manpower, the costs of operating ambulatory care centers were so great that they were usually not profitable. Likewise, many physicians were not interested in the salaried practice, and it was difficult to attract quality physicians to work in more ambulatory care centers.

Two factors worked together to make employment in ambulatory care centers more attractive. First was the beginning of the oversupply of physicians. Second, the cost of establishing or operating a medical practice, due to rising malpractice insurance costs, rose drastically.

The supply and demand of physicians is rapidly changing. In 1985 surpluses were first developing in certain physician specialties in certain geographic regions of the country. Figure 16-1 shows how the supply equaled demand in the early 1980s; since then the gap between supply and demand has been widening. As a result there will be increasing downward pressure on physicians' salaries, and the attractiveness and profitability of developing ambulatory care centers, such as urgent care centers, and comprehensive multispecialty centers by hospitals and HMOs will increase. At the same time that the supply of physicians began to exceed the demand, the cost of medical school tuition and of medical malpractice insurance premiums were skyrocketing. Many young physicians were either unable or unwilling to shoulder this heavy capitalization burden. Likewise, the steady hours and competitive salaries of ambulatory care centers were attractions to a good number of young physicians.

There have been other precedents of the movement of a self-employed professional group from self-employment to a salaried position. Some professions have made this move with relatively small reductions in income and a simultaneous increase in the prestige of their profession. For instance, the

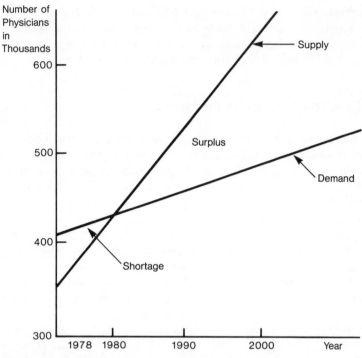

Figure 16-1 Supply and Demand of Physicians. *Source:* Report from the Graduate Advisory Committee to the Secretary of the U.S. Department of Health and Human Services, Human Resources Administration, U.S. Department of Health and Human Services, 1980.

move from individual pharmacist-owned drug stores to the drug store chains has converted many pharmacists from overworked small business persons to full-time professionals. The same is true to a lesser extent of the solo practitioner lawyer who joins a large law firm. Similar changes are also already occurring in the physician market. Many younger physicians in particular are joining HMOs as salaried physicians. Salaried physicians usually enjoy a less hectic work schedule than their solo practitioner counterparts who also must manage the business aspects of their solo practice.

Because hospitals need firm ties with ambulatory care centers to ensure rearward vertical integration hospitals will become quite active in developing ambulatory care centers. Many of these centers will probably be formed by merging solo practitioners into multiphysician ambulatory care centers, with the physicians obtaining a financial interest in the ambulatory care centers.

Another effect of the move from a shortage of physicians to a surplus of physicians will be the development of new or expanded services that employ physician manpower. Increasing use will be made of cosmetic or reconstructive surgery to improve the appearance of people who can afford these services. There also will be increased use of health and fitness evaluation, including physical checkups and health counseling. Most of the new services will be elective, with the client paying directly for the services. Many will be consumer lifestyle-driven. Physicians will also become more deeply involved in nutrition counseling, cessation of smoking clinics, sports medicine, dietary counseling, and other such services that normally are not covered by health insurance plans. All of the above services can be made available through ambulatory medical care centers and can be promoted more efficiently by the larger ambulatory care centers than by physicians in solo practice or in small group practices.

Competitiveness in Hospital Care

Prospective reimbursement systems and contracts with managed care programs, such as preferred provider organizations (PPOs), place increasing pressure on hospitals to limit expensive inpatient stays by hospital patients. The overall effect of these new pressures is to reduce the utilization of hospitals by a given population. In a geographic area with a relatively stable or slow-growing population the demand for hospital inpatient care has therefore declined significantly. For a hospital competing in this kind of market, it is imperative that it either increase its market share, reduce its scale of inpatient operations, or expand into other aspects of the health care industry.

Few hospitals are willing to decrease unilaterally their scale of operations. Most will attempt to increase their market share at the expense of direct competitors. To accomplish this goal generally requires that the hospital enhance its relationships with referring physicians and entice additional physicians to affiliate with the hospital. Active staff affiliation means that the physician will refer most of his or her patients to the hospital when acute inpatient care is deemed necessary or special testing is required.

One way of increasing the size of the active staff is to create a captive supply of affiliated physicians. This can be accomplished by the hospital engaging in rearward vertical integration through complete or partial ownership of ambulatory care centers. These ambulatory care centers can be urgent care centers or multispecialty ambulatory care centers or both. In most cases, arrangements with urgent care centers are based on referrals to staff specialists who have the responsibility of placing patients in the hospital.

Based on professional preferences among younger physicians especially, the ambulatory care industry may well be ready for a major restructuring. Those hospitals that take advantage of this will be able to remain competitive in their respective markets. Hospitals that prefer to continue the traditional hospital format will find it increasingly difficult to compete.

DEMAND FOR CONVENIENCE AMBULATORY CARE

Haley identifies two kinds of convenience freestanding medical centers.[2]

1. Centers that provide minor emergency care for minor trauma and urgent medical cases to patients on a walk-in basis. No long-term physician-patient relationship is encouraged. The primary purpose of these centers is to compete with hospital emergency rooms for their typical walk-in emergency room cases. These centers can compete successfully because they are conveniently located, and their costs and fees are much lower than the typical hospital emergency room.
2. Centers that provide the same services as the above center on a walk-in urgent care basis, but also encourage continuity of care by serving their clients on an appointment basis, especially in a primary care center.

Therefore, although the convenience medical centers were originally established to compete with the hospital emergency room, some are now competing with the traditional doctor's office as well.

For purposes of a hospital's attempts to increase hospital admissions the second type of convenience care center is clearly preferred. Too, the first type of convenience care center can be readily converted to the second type. Centers offering continuity of care, however, are politically difficult for hospitals to develop because of strong objections from community physicians. Therefore, most hospitals are not able to enter the ambulatory care business successfully.

However, hospitals should not establish convenience ambulatory care centers only for the purpose of vertical rearward integration. Probably the most important reason for doing so is that a large part of the population demands convenience medical care. Until recently they have not been able to obtain it because most ambulatory care centers operated on bankers' hours. People who work on the same type of schedule—that is, during regular daytime hours—find it difficult to arrange for appointments with a physician. Convenience medical centers provide care at times convenient to the patient.

Operating convenience ambulatory care centers can be expensive because of the long hours in which they are open—a minimum of 12 hours per day—and the double shifts of employees, including physicians, required to staff them. Therefore, it is recommended that convenience ambulatory care centers be kept small so they remain cost effective. Haley states that centers with

2,500 to 4,000 square feet of space are most cost effective.[3] The standard convenience center should consist of a waiting room, a minor trauma room, two physician offices, six examination rooms, one x-ray room, a laboratory area, two restrooms, and an administrative area. The lower the fixed over-head for operating the convenience center, the fewer will be the patient visits required to break even.

STRATEGIC PLANNING FOR AMBULATORY CARE CENTERS

Any hospital wanting to remain competitive in the future must strategically think through its options to engage in rearward vertical integration. This rearward vertical integration can be accomplished in various ways through the acquisition, partial or complete, of ambulatory care centers. Another way is to acquire or develop HMOs, especially with closed panel plans, that are largely ambulatory care centers and can funnel a considerable number of patients into the hospital. Some hospitals also may have the opportunity to merge with an existing local HMO or multispecialty ambulatory care centers. Some alternatives for rearward vertical integration are shown on Figure 16-2. Which alternative is selected is an issue that should be given much consider-

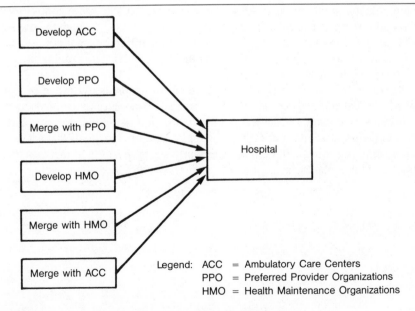

Figure 16-2 Alternative Ways To Achieve Vertical Integration

ation because it is highly dependent on the particular environment in which the hospital functions.

Because of the current restructuring of ambulatory care, hospitals must act now if they are to engage in rearward vertical integration. Reorganization, joint ventures, mergers, raising capital, and other creative approaches may be necessary. However, failure to act quickly could in the long run be more costly. Opportunities for acquisitions and mergers, already limited in most geographical locations, will diminish even further in the future.

SUMMARY

This chapter explored the vertical integration of ambulatory care facilities into hospitals. Historically, ambulatory care, notably the doctor's office, has been kept carefully separate from the hospital, especially in terms of ownership. However, the physicians who now own and control ambulatory care centers are the individuals who decide on hospital admissions and, because of their affiliation status, also determine which hospital the patient enters. Therefore, it is somewhat surprising that the vertical integration of the ambulatory care center and the hospital has not occurred earlier.

The recent restructuring of the payment method for inpatient services is dramatically changing the entire health care industry. The prospective payment method is making it imperative for hospitals to gain more control over their admission of patients. One way to accomplish this is through the ownership or at least control of physician's actions regarding hospital admissions. In this way hospitals can be assured that their hospital bed utilization remains high enough to ensure profitability.

Two issues make it particularly opportune for hospitals to engage in rearward vertical integration. The first is the increasing surplus of physicians, especially in certain specialties. Second is the increasing demand of a large part of the population for convenient ambulatory care. Hospitals that act early to integrate rearward will be in a particularly strong position to increase their market share at the expense of those hospitals that fail to act decisively.

NOTES

1. M. Haley, "Positioning Doctors for Convenience Medicine," *ACHA/Journal* 29, no. 4 (July/August 1984):95–110.

2. Ibid.

3. Ibid.

Chapter 17

Strategic Development Planning for Health Maintenance Organizations: Application of CPM-PERT

HIGHLIGHTS

- The CPM-PERT Project Planning Process
- The IPA Physician Organization and Contractual Process
- The HMO Marketing Process
- Activities Required to Develop IPA-HMO Financial Plan
- Summary

17

Health maintenance organizations (HMOs) have been in existence since the first Kaiser Permanente prepaid health care plans were developed shortly after World War II. However, except for one isolated prepaid plan in New York City and others in California, HMOs really did not gain momentum until President Nixon signed into law the HMO Act of 1973. With this act the federal government went on record as supporting the development of HMOs through funding feasibility planning and initial development and through the provision of government guarantees on startup loans to new HMOs.

The initial impact of the law was minimal. Although there was much interest and enthusiasm for developing HMOs, professional staff to develop prepaid plans were scarce and inexperienced. In addition the federal government imposed considerable controls on any feasibility and planning grants to ensure that federal funds would not be wasted.

As a result, the planning and development activities of early HMOs that were funded by federal grants were slow and frequently painful and disappointing. However, the process of doing feasibility studies, planning, and initial development evolved into a well-organized planning process in which many individuals were trained. What finally emerged was a well-established system for screening HMO proposals. Another result was the development of professional planning teams that produced HMO development plans according to a general process and model developed over a long period of time using trial and error. There was a wide dissemination of the HMO planning processes thus producing many qualified HMO planners.

Although not all HMOs that were developed during the initial years of the HMO planning process survived, many still exist today and prove the viability of the HMO in the American health care system. They laid a foundation for today's rapid growth of HMOs. Initially, by government edict, all prospective HMOs qualifying for federal grants had to be not-for-profit. This, in retrospect, was an unfortunate decision because developing HMOs are in

221

constant need of capital, and not-for-profit organizations usually find it more difficult to raise capital than for-profit organizations. In the 1980s, the federal government began to realize this fact and encouraged for-profit organizations to enter the HMO field. Since then, the major source of growth in HMOs has come from for-profit organizations, especially large national indemnity insurance companies.

This chapter reviews the approaches and processes used for the feasibility study, planning, and initial development stages of HMOs. These approaches are quite structured and reflect a proven method of general feasibility and planning for health care organizations in general.

There are two major types of HMOs. The first is the closed panel plan that employs its own staff physicians and owns its own ambulatory medical care centers. Some closed panel models contract with an established group practice of physicians. The second type is the independent practice association (IPA) or open panel plan that utilizes independent physicians who practice from their own offices and are organized as an IPA. The IPA in turn contracts with the HMO to provide physician services. Because the vast majority of new HMOs are of the IPA model, this chapter focuses on that model.

A project planning process is described below and then applied to HMO planning activities for physician organization, HMO marketing, and HMO financial management.

CPM-PERT PROJECT PLANNING PROCESS

A technique used in planning and scheduling the various planning activities is the critical path method (CPM), also called the project evaluation and review technique (PERT). Although, some authors claim that the two techniques differ to some extent, over time the differences have blurred, and the combined technique is commonly referred to as CPM-PERT, a project planning technique.

CPM-PERT allows one to arrange and schedule any number of sequential or simultaneous activities with the aid of a network model. All the planner needs to do is identify and specify the activity, estimate the time needed for the activity to be completed in its entirety, and determine which activities need to be completed before the subsequent activities can be started. Activities that need to be completed just before a given activity can be started are termed predecessor activities.

Table 17–1 lists seven activities, identified by the numbers 1 to 7. The seven activities are connected by nodes and events that are separately numbered as shown in Figure 17-1. For instance, activity 1, which takes 5 weeks to complete, is connected by events 1 and 2. Activity 2 takes 8 weeks and is

Table 17-1 Example of List of Activities for CPM-PERT Application

Activity	Time in Weeks	Predecessor Activity
1	5	—
2	8	—
3	7	1
4	4	2
5	3	1
6	5	3,4
7	8	3,4
8	0	5,6

connected by events 1 and 3. Activity 3 takes 7 weeks, is connected by events 2 and 4, and cannot be started until activity 1 is completed. Activities 6 and 7, connected by events 4 and 5 and 4 and 6, respectively, require the completion of activities 3 and 4 before they can be started. Activity 8 is a dummy activity. It requires no time to be completed. It only shows that activities 5 and 6 must be completed before the entire project is finished. The critical path in the project follows the events 1-3-4-6 and takes 21 weeks. Within the 21-week time limit all other activities can be completed.

THE IPA PHYSICIAN ORGANIZATION AND CONTRACTUAL PROCESS

The most critical part in forming an IPA-HMO is the organization of a large group of physicians into an IPA. The IPA must contain a sufficient

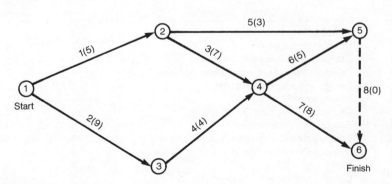

Note: Time to complete activity in weeks is shown in parentheses.

Figure 17-1 CPM-PERT Diagram for Example Problem

number of physicians in all primary medical care areas and ideally in all secondary medical care areas. Tertiary medical care can usually be negotiated separately and does not need to be represented in the IPA medical specialty composition.

The first IPA development activity in a community is always the most difficult because physicians must first be educated about its purpose and the benefits of membership. The new HMO product will not bring patients to the physician immediately, so the physician must have implicit trust that not only is the organization worthwhile but that the HMO concept will also be "bought" by the community. This sales job is difficult and time consuming. If there is an HMO already in the marketplace, the organization of the IPA is made easier by the desire of the target physicians not to lose market share.

The steps required to organize an IPA and the approximate time needed to perform each of the 14 activities are shown in Table 17-2. Note that some of the activities are quite lengthy and must be done ahead of others, whereas other pairs of activities can be done simultaneously. Again, the times for each step must be adjusted according to how well the HMO concept is established in your community.

To determine the overall time required to perform all necessary activities related to the IPA organization process, a CPM-PERT network has been developed, as shown in Figure 17-2. It shows the order in which each of the 14 activities must be performed. It also identifies the critical or bottleneck path. This path determines what the earliest date is by which the entire project can be completed; in this case the date is 52 weeks. All other activities can also be completed within this time span.

Table 17-2 Activities Required to Develop an IPA-HMO Physician Organization Project

Activity	Activity Description	Time in Weeks	Predecessor Activity
1	Contact physician organizations in area	6	—
2	Develop physician risk sharing	10	1
3	Establish IPA steering committee	8	1
4	Develop physician compensation package	4	2
5	Design and print IPA brochure	7	2
6	Incorporate IPA	9	3
7	Develop contracts for IPA physicians	9	4
8	Run physician fee survey	5	4
9	Educate area physicians about IPA	13	5
10	Develop IPA-HMO contract	6	6
11	Dummy activity	0	7
12	Obtain letters of intent to join IPA	8	8,9,11
13	Develop IPA policies for referral and utilization	9	10
14	Sign up IPA physicians	4	12,13
15	Train physician office staffs	4	14

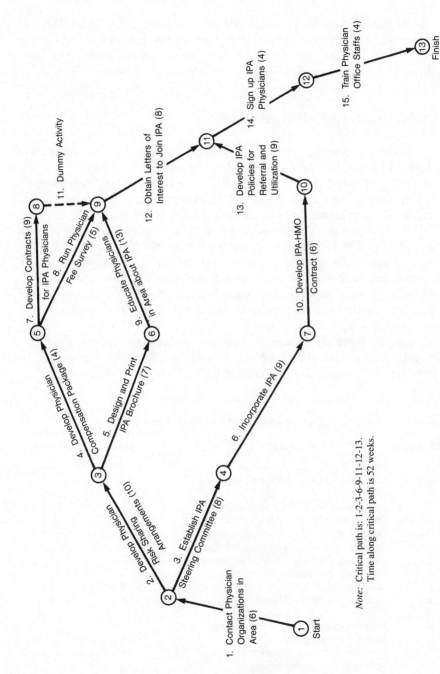

Figure 17-2 CPM-PERT Chart for IPA-HMO Physician Organization Project

Note: Critical path is: 1-2-3-6-9-11-12-13.
Time along critical path is 52 weeks.

Many hospitals and hospital networks are establishing IPA model HMOs in order to create a captive audience of physicians who are already tied into the referral network and who have communication links in place. It is quite obvious that in such cases the critical path is much shortened.

THE HMO MARKETING PROCESS

An HMO needs physicians to function. However, without a sufficient number of members, the fixed cost of operation would quickly drive it into bankruptcy. It is therefore important that a new IPA-HMO increase its membership as quickly as possible to the breakeven level. To accomplish this requires the development of a sound strategic marketing plan.

Table 17-3 lists the 15 activities required to develop the marketing plan for the IPA-HMO. Note that the first step required is to recruit and train marketing staff to complement the executive staff. Before the marketing effort can be started the details of the health care benefit package must be determined. At the same time as those details are determined, employers can be contacted, promotional materials can be developed, and initial monthly enrollment projections can be determined.

From that point on employees must be contacted so that group contract negotiations can take place, and final monthly enrollment projections can be prepared. Also employee promotional materials must be developed, and a

Table 17-3 Activities Required to Develop an IPA-HMO Marketing Plan

Activity	Activity Description	Time Required in Weeks	Predecessor Activity
1	Recruit and train marketing staff	5	—
2	Complete details of health care benefit package	3	1
3	Organize community outreach activities	10	1
4	Contact employees in service area	6	1
5	Develop employer promotional package	3	1
6	Prepare initial monthly enrollment projections	4	2,4
7	Implement employer promotional package	4	5
8	Undertake employer group contract negotiations	8	6,7
9	Develop employer promotional materials	6	6,7
10	Finalize employer group contracts	6	8
11	Print employee promotional materials	3	9
12	Select employer groups	16	10,11
13	Organize health care symposium	16	3
14	Hold health care symposium	2	13
15	Prepare final monthly enrollment projections	2	10,11

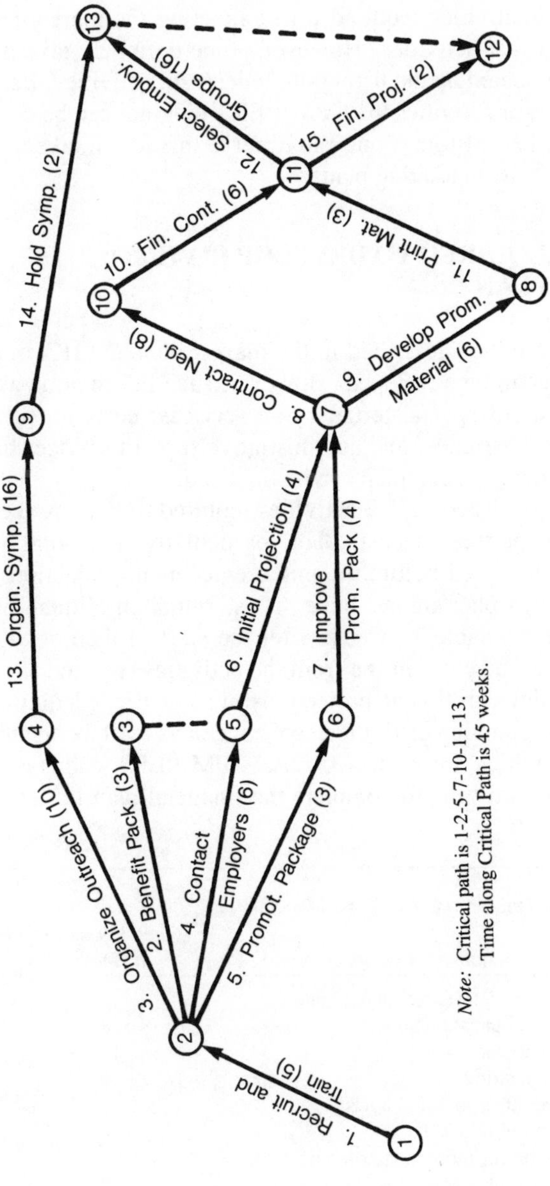
1
2
3
4
5
6
7
8
9
10
11
12
13
1. Recruit and Train (5)
3. Organize Outreach (10)
2. Benefit Pack. (3)
4. Contact Employers (6)
5. Promot. Package (3)
6. Initial Projection (4)
7. Improve Prom. Pack (4)
8. Contract Neg. (8)
9. Develop Prom. Material (6)
10. Fin. Cont. (6)
11. Print Mat. (3)
12. Select Employ. Groups (16)
13. Organ. Symp. (16)
14. Hold Symp. (2)
15. Fin. Proj. (2)

Note: Critical path is 1-2-5-7-10-11-13.
Time along Critical Path is 45 weeks.

Figure 17-3 CPM-PERT Chart for IPA-HMO Marketing Plan

health care symposium must be organized to publicize the IPA-HMO that is under development.

Most of the 15 activities required for completing the marketing plan are interrelated with other activities. However, some definitely take precedence over others, as indicated by the listing of predecessor activities. Based on this listing of predecessor activities the CPM-PERT diagram can be developed as shown on Figure 17-3. From it one can observe that it will take a total of 45 weeks to complete the marketing plan.

ACTIVITIES REQUIRED TO DEVELOP IPA-HMO FINANCIAL PLAN

Based on the activities described in the market plan and IPA organization the financial plan can be developed. However, such information as hospitalization costs, costs of special tertiary care services, costs for allied health services, costs for insurance, and administrative support services must all be estimated before the financial plan can be finalized.

On Table 17-4 are listed the 12 activities required to prepare the financial plan. The details of the financial plan, particularly the monthly revenue flows, cannot be finalized before the initial enrollment projections prepared as part of the market plan are available. These initial enrollment projections will only become available 15 weeks after the start of the overall planning activities. However, as you can see from the activities required for the financial plan, the initial enrollment projections are not needed until 19 weeks after the start of planning activities, so no delays will be incurred. The financial plan activities are projected on a CPM-PERT chart as shown on Figure 17-4. The total time to complete the financial plan in this case is 39 weeks.

Table 17-4 Activities Required to Develop Financial Plan

Activity	Activity Description	Time Required in Weeks	Predecessor Activity
1	Prepare administration cost estimates	12	—
2	Collect local utilization statistics	8	—
3	Collect local cost statistics	10	—
4	Do actuarial study	9	2,3
5	Prepare monthly revenue flows	5	4
6	Prepare monthly cost flows	4	4
7	Prepare monthly income statements	6	1,5,6
8	Prepare monthly cash flows	7	1,5,6
9	Prepare annual income statements	4	7,8
10	Prepare annual balance sheets	3	7,8
11	Prepare loan repayment schedule	4	9,10
12	Prepare adverse condition analysis	6	7

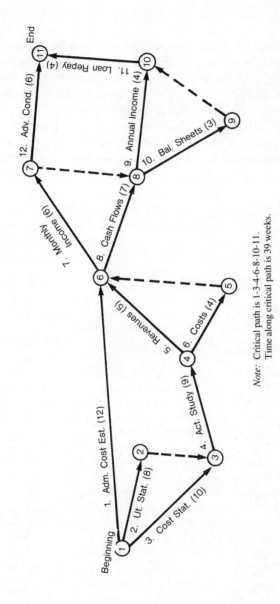

Note: Critical path is 1-3-4-6-8-10-11.
Time along critical path is 39 weeks.

Figure 17-4 CPM-PERT Chart for IPA-HMO Financial Plan

SUMMARY

This chapter presented two case approaches to developing the initial startup plans for an IPA-HMO. However, these approaches do not comprise the complete set of strategic planning activities for an IPA-HMO or, for that matter, for any HMO. Strategic planning for operational HMOs requires the same strategic planning process described earlier in this book.

To ensure that the planning activities can be completed in a timely manner, a project planning tool called CPM-PERT was utilized. This tool ensures that the sequential nature and predecessor nature of certain activities are explicitly considered.

Chapter 18

Strategic Management in Home Health Care Organizations

HIGHLIGHTS

- Defining the Home Health Care Market
- Opportunities in the Home Health Care Market
- Home Health Care Clients
- Home Health Care As an Alternative to Nursing Homes
- Future Growth in Home Health Care
- Summary

232

18

One of the health care industries that has rapidly developed during the past 10 years, especially in terms of number of firms involved, is the home health care industry. Reasons for its rapid development are the low entry barrier into the marketplace, the increased demand for home health care, the low level of regulation of the industry, and the minimal qualifications required to provide the service. As this industry reaches a more mature stage in its life cycle, these factors will change to resemble other health care industries. In most states in the late 1980s, just about any businessperson can begin offering home health care services with home health aides who have received minimal training, usually from experienced and licensed nurses. Most likely the businessperson will hire a registered nurse to be the director of services and director of training. That simple staff structure will satisfy almost all the entry requirements for the home health care business in most states. To receive direct Medicare and Medicaid reimbursement the agency will need to meet other requirements and regulations, but most startup firms prefer to concentrate on the more lucrative and less regulated private-fee-for-service market.

This chapter examines the opportunities in home health care, especially for established health care organizations, such as hospitals, nursing homes, and HMOs. It also discusses who the home health care clients are and reviews the cost effectiveness of health care in relation to the alternatives of hospitalization and nursing home institutionalization. Finally, the future growth of home health care is considered. This growth will make home health care an attractive industry for new entrepreneurs to enter. Yet, an attractive industry will also attract the more experienced and stronger financed companies. Health industry growth also attracts greater regulation and liability issues as well. All of these factors will combine to create a very different health care industry in 1995.

DEFINING THE HOME HEALTH CARE MARKET

As a whole the home health care industry provides services to individuals and families in their places of residence for the purpose of promoting, maintaining, and restoring health or minimizing the effects of illness and disability.

There is a tendency to think of the home health care market in terms of traditional home health care provided by the Visiting Nurses Association (VNA). The VNA has and continues to provide skilled home nursing services, occupational and physical therapy services, and social work services. As a not-for-profit organization the VNA tries to provide services where the need is greatest. Its main financial concern is to break even or, if losses are incurred, to cover those losses with gifts or subsidies.

In the classification of home health care the VNA is considered a staffing organization. A staffing agency is a home health care organization that provides nurses and other allied health personnel for a fee wherever a need is indicated. VNAs and other traditional home health agencies are now moving, through corporate reorganization, into the relatively new areas of home health that are described below.

The next most prevalent home health care organization is the distributor—through sales, rental, or leasing—of durable medical equipment, such as hospital beds, wheelchairs, oxygen equipment, etc. A third type of home health care organization is one that provides special "high tech" services, such as intravenous nutritional feeding services and home dialysis. Meals on Wheels could fit into that category as well. The fourth and last type of home health care organization is essentially a supplier or retailer of self-care products, including diagnostic equipment, such as pregnancy kits, colorectal cancer detection kits, blood pressure analyzers, and the like.

OPPORTUNITIES IN THE HOME HEALTH CARE MARKET

From the point of view of continuity of care, one could argue that the hospital is in an ideal position to engage in forward vertical integration into home health care. A home health care staffing organization seems at first to be the most logical type of home health service for a hospital to develop. It provides continuity of care and is most compatible with the typical hospital services. However, home health care staffing is very labor intensive and also very competitive, because of the low barriers of entry into the home health care staffing market. Because of the high level of competition in this field, a hospital may find it more beneficial to consider entering into contractual arrangements with existing home health care staffing organizations to provide home health care services for its patients. One other problem with the home health care staffing model is the extensive level of training required for the home health care nurses and aides. Especially considering the liability issues that already affect hospitals, the limited supervision that can be provided to home health care personnel increases liability risks drastically, causing even greater costs for training and recruitment.

Developing a distributorship for durable medical equipment is another alternate home health care organization that a hospital can develop. Because most of the equipment supplied by such a distributor is also used in the hospital, acquiring a distributorship seems to be a logical way to engage in forward vertical integration. From a management point of view it is probably a more desirable area to move into than a home health care staffing organization. However, the medical equipment distribution market is also very competitive because of its relatively low entry barriers. In addition this market lends itself very well to franchising. A franchise organization has the benefits of mass purchasing and economies of scale in advertising.

The specialized services company in the home health care industry is also ideally suited for forward vertical integration. Again the services provided are already being used in hospitals, and as a result required expertise is not new to the hospital. Technical expertise can be offered by the hospital's physicians. The most difficult aspect of developing high-tech home health care is convincing the discharge planners and physicians that the formerly hospital-only services can be provided in a quality manner at home. Another problem is the general lack of third party reimbursement, including private insurance, for high-tech services. High-tech home care is generally a high-priced, fee-for-service program. This factor limits the total pool of patients available from a given hospital.

The well-managed hospital that is in good financial condition and is interested in forward vertical integration may well consider a strategic move into all three home health care businesses. Most general hospitals have at least some expertise in each one of the services that the home health care agencies provide. If a hospital decides to enter into any one or all three home health care businesses, it would most likely establish a separate management organization for each one. The home health care staffing organizations make the most sense in terms of providing continuity of care, whereas the distributorship and high-tech home care make the most sense because of the expertise the hospital has in providing the respective services. Hospitals should match the type of home health care they plan to provide with the types of diagnoses that are likely to be discharged to that service. Many hospitals have organized multiple home health services organizations to serve the needs of different patient populations. A hospital network with a well-established and respected name would potentially be at a competitive advantage over other agencies with relatively new or unknown names, qualifications, and reputations. The above opportunities are visually portrayed in Figure 18-1.

HOME HEALTH CARE CLIENTS

The most important target clientele for home health care is the age group of persons 65 years and older. This age cohort is also the most rapidly growing segment of the American population and is expected to continue its growth until 2050. More specifically, the age group 75–84 years seems to have a very high rate of use of home health care because members of this group remain fairly independent in their homes. Although the senior group currently makes up about 11 percent of the population, they account for 29 percent of all health care expenditures (Figure 18-2). The elderly also enter hospitals twice as often and stay twice as long as the general population. It is therefore not surprising that whenever home health care is mentioned one immediately thinks of senior adults. Also, the notion that long-term home health care, a relatively new service, is an alternative to nursing home care has strengthened the linkage of home health care to the elderly. Therefore, when discussing home health care, a greater emphasis is placed on the 65 and older age group, even though the terminally ill child, the disabled, and the

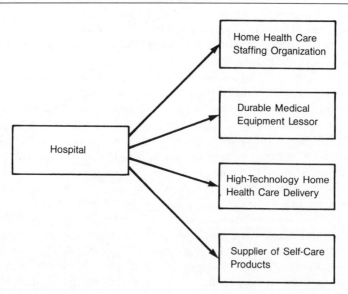

Figure 18-1 Opportunities for Hospitals To Engage in Forward Vertical Integration

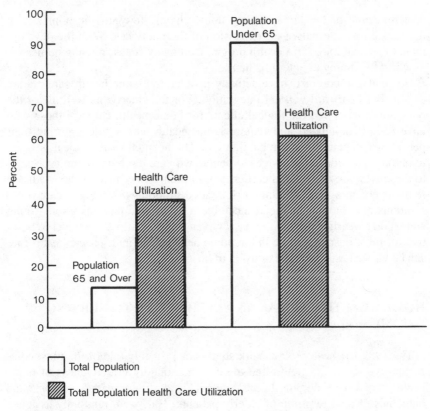

Figure 18-2 Health Care Utilization of 65 and Over versus Those Under 65

physically and mentally handicapped are also in need of home health care services.

Much debate and discussion about the cost effectiveness of home health care versus nursing home care has still not resolved the issue. Most very ill or very old and disabled people are more easily and better cared for in a skilled nursing facility (highest level of nursing home care). Yet, there are also many elderly people in health-related facilities (lower level of health care) and in intermediate care facilities who could quite easily live at home with adequate home health care. However, home health care is usually only feasible if the sick elderly person has someone living with her or him. In that case home health care is probably the most cost-effective alternative to nursing home care.

One would expect that many nursing homes would have been horizontally integrated to provide both institutional and home health care. However, except for some of the large nursing home chains, few nursing homes have developed this alternative for expansion of their services. With the development of special long-term health programs in many states, nursing homes are now just beginning to enter this market.

Hospitals, in contrast, have actively invaded the home health care market as a form of forward vertical integration. For the elderly, as well as for the population under 65, the logical clients for home health care are those who have been hospitalized and require home health care services during their period of recuperation and rehabilitation. The hospital is in an ideal position to market its home care services to people who are discharged and especially to those who are discharged earlier than in the past because of the Medicare reimbursement system of diagnostic-related groupings. Managed care organizations also have a financial incentive to discharge patients—both young and elderly—earlier than in the past. Given this scenario it is almost imperative for most hospitals to be in the home health care field. Home health care can be viewed as a natural extension of hospital care.

HOME HEALTH CARE AS AN ALTERNATIVE TO NURSING HOMES

The 1982 Rochester, New York study was probably one of the most comprehensive studies to determine the cost and quality effectiveness of home health care versus nursing home care.[1] This study compared the costs and outcomes of a large group of elderly patients. Half were randomly assigned to receive frequent health evaluations, including home health care by a health care team consisting of a physician, nurse, and social worker. The other half of the patients were the control group and were treated only as required. Before being randomly assigned, both experimental and control group patients were interviewed to determine their suitability to take part in the study. The experimental and control groups were generally comparable with regard to most demographic characteristics, previous health care utilization, diagnoses, and in the scores of questionnaires administered prior to the study.

The results of the study indicated that there was no significant difference in cost of care between the surviving members of the experimental group and the surviving members of the control group. The cost statistics as shown on Table 18-1 indicate that the experimental group's in-home added cost for its surviving members was virtually identical to the control group's out-of-home cost for its surviving members.

A number of other studies have attempted to show that home health care cost is lower than nursing home care cost, but only a very few used a comparable control population as in the Rochester study. The problem with

Table 18-1 Cost Comparison of Experimental Group and Control Group Patients After 3 Months

Patients (n)	Out-of-Home Day Cost	In-Home Day Cost	Total Day Cost
PATIENTS WHO DIED			
Experimental group (21)	$ 57.67	$34.91	$ 92.58
Control group (16)	110.79	13.87	124.66
Total (37)	80.64	25.81	106.45
SURVIVORS			
Experimental group (60)	9.83	21.99	31.82
Control group (59)	16.19	16.41	32.61
Total (119)	12.99	19.22	32.21

Source: "Randomized Trial of a Team Approach to Home Care" by A. Groth-Juncker et al., University of Rochester School of Medicine and Dentistry, 1982.

many of these studies is that the two populations compared may be significantly different. A Transamerica-Occidental Life study showed that inpatient hospital care for a terminal cancer patient for 18 days would cost $19,450, whereas hospice care at home would cost $723.[2] An Aetna Life and Casualty study showed that a baby born with breathing and feeding problems could be cared for at home with home health care support for one-third of the cost of hospitalization, and a quadraplegic individual could be cared for at home at slightly half the cost of hospitalization.[3] In both cases, of course, someone would need to be at home to provide routine care for both patients. Any potential cost associated with this caregiver was not included in the home health care cost figures.

Because of the above confounding studies, one can conclude that the appropriate level of health care in some cases may be in-home care, but in many other cases the institutional setting is the appropriate place. New services, such as long-term home health care, will develop and expand to meet more effectively the needs of the patients who are not well served by the traditional modes of care.

FUTURE GROWTH IN HOME HEALTH CARE

Although the question whether home health care is more cost effective than institutionalized care, especially for nursing home patients, is still unanswered, there is little doubt about the recent and continued growth in home health care. This growth presents considerable opportunities not only for new entrepreneurs but also for existing health care organizations. The most logical organizations to expand into home health care are the hospitals. However, one may wonder, why have nursing homes been reluctant so far? After all, most home health care and nursing care are provided postacutely, and the two types of organizations often vie for the same patients.

Predicasts, a marketing research firm, predicts that home health care revenues will reach $12.2 billion in 1988 and $24.8 billion in 1995.[4] Considering that 1983 home health care revenues amount to $6.3 billion, it is clear that growth is considerable. Figure 18-3 shows graphically the magnitude of the projected growth. The rapid growth of home health care is, however, not going to be profitable for all concerned. Many of the smaller firms will face increasing difficulty in competing, especially if more hospitals with their built-in clientele and their extensive experience in patient care move more aggressively into the home health care field.

With the growth in home health care, regulation of the quality of care will become stricter and certification of home health care will be increasingly required. This change by itself will improve the quality of care, but also raise its cost. It will also severely limit the availability of qualified personnel, thus increasing the difficulty of small firms in competing against the larger and more established home health care organizations owned or affiliated with hospitals, nursing homes, and HMOs.

SUMMARY

One can view the home health care industry as consisting of four segments. The largest and most prominent segment is the home health care staffing organization. Next is the supplier and distributor of medical equipment. Then comes the supplier of high-technology services, such as nutritional feeding, home dialysis, and electronic monitoring. Finally, there is the supplier of self-care products, such as diagnostic testing.

Although the last two home health care segments at present are the smallest they potentially may have the most explosive growth. Both segments lend themselves to the development of new products and services, and history reveals that useful products and high-technology services find a ready market. The self-care products segment has an especially great potential because the potential market is the entire population, not just the sick.

Opportunities abound in all four home health care segments. The best-situated groups to participate in this market are the health care organizations, such as hospitals, who have a solid and good reputation. They have the customer contacts as well because much of home care is needed following hospitalization. Because home health care requires a separate organization and management many of the voluntary sector hospitals may be unwilling to move aggressively into that market. However, nearly all for-profit hospitals will do so, viewing it as a potentially lucrative form of forward vertical integration.

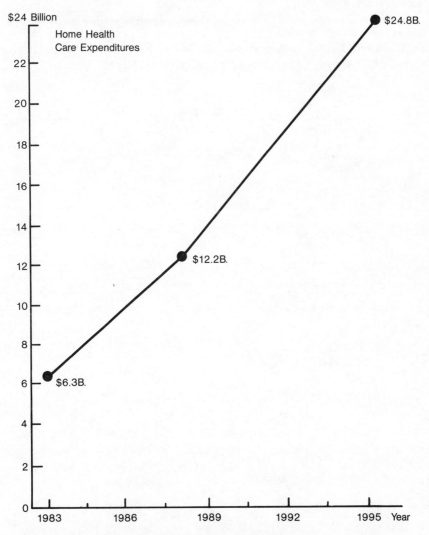

Figure 18-3 Projected Growth of Home Health Care Expenditures. *Source: Hospitals,* Vol. 59, p. 64, American Hospital Publishing Company, © May 16, 1985.

NOTES

1. A. Groth-Juncker, J. G. Zimmer, J. McCusker, and T. F. Williams, "Randomized Trial of a New Team Approach to Home Care," Research report, University of Rochester School of Medicine and Dentistry, 1982, 3–19.

2. "Home Health Care Saves Everyone a Bundle," *National Underwriter-Life and Health Edition,* March 29, 1985, p. 10.

3. "The Insurers' Big Push for Home Health Care," *Business Week,* May 28, 1984, p. 128.

4. "Home Care Agencies Up 25 Percent Since 1984," *Hospitals,* May 16,1985, p. 64.

Part VII

Strategic Management and Its Future Impacts

The first chapter in this part, Chapter 19, explores the problems, issues, and opportunities for multihospital or multi-institutional systems. The growth of multi-institutional systems has been rapid and is anticipated to continue. Numerous independent hospitals will elect to join multi-institutional systems because of the expertise, technology, management specialization, economies of scale, and purchasing advantages that the multi-institutional system provides.

Chapter 20 discusses the impact of prospective case payment mechanisms, such as diagnostic-related groups (DRGs). DRGs do, and will increasingly in the future, shorten lengths of stays in the hospital and thus lower hospital occupancy rates. The primary way that hospitals will be able to increase their inpatient occupancy rates is by taking market share away from other hospitals. The resulting strategies will include active competition for physician affiliations and engaging in vertical integration by acquiring or developing ambulatory care centers, home health agencies, and HMOs. The inpatient orientation of hospitals will weaken as they become competitors in nonacute settings.

Chapter 21 addresses the issue of how a hospital can compete in the new competitive environment. The need to seize the competitive initiative is emphasized. Act; do not wait until you have to react. The second issue addressed is mistakes made in strategic planning. This chapter identifies some of the many pitfalls that the reader should avoid.

The fourth and final chapter in Part VII, Chapter 22, discusses the issues associated with strategy implementation. One of the important and necessary requirements for successful strategy implementation is the active participation by lower and middle-level management in the strategic planning process.

Chapter 19

Multi-Institutional Systems

HIGHLIGHTS

- History and Background
- Forces Encouraging Independent Hospitals To Join Multi-Institutional Systems
- New Developments in Multi-Institutional Systems
- Strategic Management of Multi-Institutional Systems
- Summary

19

The concept of multi-institutional systems in health care dates back some 50 years. It has not been until the past 10 to 15 years, however, that there has been a rapid increase in the number of multi-institutional systems. In 1984 about 32 percent of community hospitals and about 36 percent of community hospital beds were part of multi-institutional arrangements. This movement toward multi-institutional systems is projected to accelerate so that by 1990 close to 60 percent of all acute care hospitals and about 40 percent of acute care hospital beds will be aligned with a multi-institutional system.

This trend is fueled by individual hospital's concern for survival and growth amid drastic changes in the environment affecting the hospital industry. Multi-institutional systems, applying management theory and techniques and utilizing economies of scale, can adapt well to the increasingly complex and volatile health care environment. This environment imposes pressures related to operating costs, maintenance of quality service, financial capacity, reimbursement, and many other factors that make survival an issue of considerable concern.

HISTORY AND BACKGROUND

Multi-institutional systems can be divided into two general categories: (1) investor-owned, for profit systems and (2) not-for-profit, voluntary systems, including both secular and religious affiliated systems. The hospital industry in the early 1900s was dominated by proprietary hospitals that were usually owned by a group of physicians. The passage of the federal Hill-Burton legislation in 1946, however, made available to communities matching federal funds to finance the construction of new hospitals. As a result, many small physician-owned hospitals were replaced by larger, more sophisticated, voluntary not-for-profit institutions. The percentage of investor-

247

owned hospitals decreased from 56 percent in 1910 to under 16 percent in 1969. A shortage of capital and an inability to compete effectively with publicly financed facilities forced many proprietary hospitals out of business.

A significant change in the trend toward publicly financed hospitals occurred with the introduction of Medicare and Medicaid legislation in 1965. Federal money flowing into hospital coffers enticed many new for-profit hospital corporations to start up operations. With that entry into the hospital field, the new move toward corporate ownership and management of American hospitals began.

In the late 1960s, for-profit hospital corporations limited their acquisitions to hospitals that were in financial difficulty. In the early 1970s, companies began constructing their own hospitals, primarily in the Sunbelt states where an expanding population base, minimal union activity, and fewer state regulations created an attractive, more profitable environment. In the mid-1970s, however, when market conditions weakened, interest rates rose, and inflation increased the cost of construction materials, for-profit hospital chains began concentrating on hospital management contracts as an alternative to additional hospital ownership to avoid the large capital investments required for continuing expansion.

Not-for-profit hospitals, in contrast, have been drawn toward multi-institutional systems for slightly different reasons. Although both not-for-profit and for-profit hospitals face the same adverse environmental factors, not-for-profit hospitals have looked to reorganization as a way of preserving their religious or voluntary traditions, increasing services offered, and ensuring long-term survival.

In 1981, not-for-profit multihospital systems, including religious-affiliated systems, comprised about 20 percent of the hospitals and about 26 percent of hospital beds. Investor-owned multihospital systems comprised about 13 percent of hospitals and about 10 percent of hospital beds, as shown in Figure 19-1.

Although investor-owned multihospital systems comprise only about 13 percent of all hospitals, those systems tend to be larger than not-for-profit hospital systems, including religious affiliated systems. Investor-owned systems average 24 hospitals and over 3100 beds per system as compared to nonprofit systems, which average five hospitals and over 1100 beds per system (Figure 19-2). Of all hospitals and beds in multi-institutional systems, investor-owned systems contain about 40 percent of all system hospitals representing about 28 percent of all system beds, as shown in Figure 19-3. The percentage of hospitals that are part of multi-institutional systems is expected to continue to increase at a rate of 5-7 percent per year, whereas the percentage of hospital beds in such systems is expected to grow at a rate of 3 to 4 percent each year.

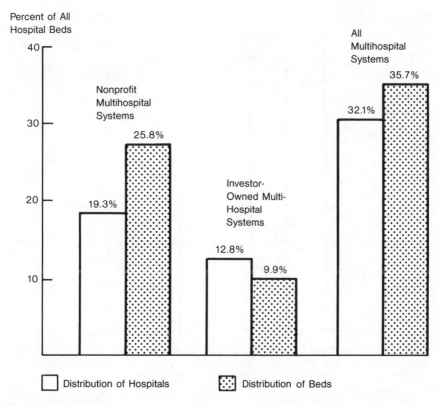

Figure 19-1 Distribution of Hospitals and Beds for Multihospital Systems in 1981. *Source: Health Progress* (formerly *Hospital Progress*), pp. 48–53, Catholic Health Association of the United States, © April 1983.

A survey of multihospital systems for 1983 as reported by Johnson reveals that there is an amazing similarity in hospital size between investor-owned and secular nonprofit multihospital systems.[1] The largest hospitals are found in public multihospital systems. Of the 179 multihospital systems surveyed, which included over 1900 hospitals, the average hospital had 166 beds, as shown in Table 19-1.

The 1983 survey of 147 multihospital systems also showed that after-tax return on revenues was substantially higher for the investor-owned multihospital systems (6.57 percent) than for the secular nonprofit systems (3.65 percent). The latter figure was also tax free. The return on revenues figure was nearly identical for the Catholic and other religious nonprofit multihospital systems; it was 4.60 and 4.65 percent, respectively, as shown in Table 19-2.

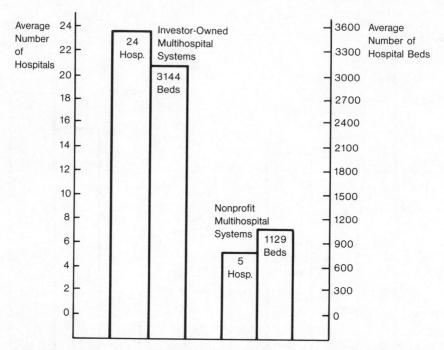

Figure 19-2 Comparison of Average Number of Hospitals and Average Number of Beds per Multihospital System in 1981. *Source: Health Progress* (formerly *Hospital Progress*), pp. 48–53, Catholic Health Association of the United States, © April 1983.

The five largest multihospital systems on the basis of total hospitals operated worldwide and total beds operated worldwide are shown on Table 19-3. Note that one of the largest investor-owned multi-hospital systems, Hospital Corporation of America, operates more beds than the next four largest systems combined.

Table 19-1 Numbers of Hospitals and Beds for Multihospital Systems in 1983

Type of Systems	Number of Systems	Number of Hospitals	Number of Beds	Hospitals per System	Beds per System	Beds per Hospital
Investor-owned	30	869	123,810	29.0	4127	143
Secular, nonprofit	85	583	86,266	6.9	1015	148
Catholic, nonprofit	27	230	53,077	8.5	1966	231
Other religious, nonprofit	23	185	34,749	8.0	1511	188
Public	14	49	20,648	3.5	1475	421
Total	179	1916	318,550	10.7	1780	166

Source: Modern Healthcare, pp. 65–84, Crain Communications Inc., © May 15, 1984.

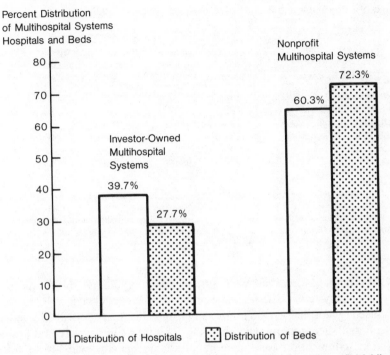

Figure 19-3 Distribution of Hospitals and Beds for Investor-Owned and Nonprofit Multihospi-tal Systems in 1981. *Source: Health Progress* (formerly *Hospital Progress*), pp. 48–53, Catho-lic Health Association of the United States, © April 1983.

FORCES ENCOURAGING INDEPENDENT HOSPITALS TO JOIN MULTI-INSTITUTIONAL SYSTEMS

The movement toward multi-institutional systems is not a phenomenon that has occurred overnight. Public policy generally encourages coordination among hospitals and the development of integrated regional hospital systems as a way of improving access, comprehensiveness, and continuity of care; of gaining economies of scale; of reducing duplication; and of improving quality. Also, independent hospitals make easier targets than more powerful multi-institutional systems when the regional and state planning agencies try to reduce excess hospital beds by pressuring hospitals to close or combine with larger hospitals or hospital systems.

Table 19-2 Revenues and Profits for Multihospital Systems in 1983

Type of Systems	Number of Systems	Revenues* (millions of dollars)	Profits† (millions of dollars)	Average Profit per System (millions of dollars)	Return on Revenues (%)
Investor-owned	20	$11131	$ 731	$43	6.57
Secular, nonprofit	72	10078	368	6	3.65
Catholic, nonprofit	24	5678	261	12	4.60
Other religious, nonprofit	18	3358	156	9	4.65
Public	13	3235	−235	−21	−7.26
Total	147	33480	1281	9	3.83

* Gross Revenues or charges plus bad debt and minus discounts taken by Medicare, Medicaid, Blue Cross, etc.
† From continuing operations, not including gifts. Investor-owned systems show after-tax profits.
Source: Modern Healthcare, pp. 65–84, Crain Communications Inc., © May 15, 1984.

Other market forces as well are encouraging the trend toward multi-institutional systems. The financial problems and capital acquisition difficulties faced by hospitals in the mid-1980s will be further aggravated by reduced federal and state government financing for care of the elderly and poor. In addition, competition for the more profitable patients will create further financial and occupancy problems for the weaker hospitals who do not have the status or capability of attracting these patients. Changes in medical practice will also occur as patients are moved from expensive inpatient care to alternative and lower-cost ambulatory care or home health care. Also, aggressive development and growth strategies by nonprofit systems may

Table 19-3 The Five Largest Multihospital Systems in Terms of Beds in 1983

	Beds			Hospitals		
	U.S.	Foreign	Worldwide	U.S.	Foreign	Worldwide
1. Hospital Corporation of America	53,754	2,472	56,226	366	24	390
2. Humana, Inc.	17,365	465	17,830	87	3	90
3. American Medical	10,744	3,530	14,274	78	26	104
4. National Medical Enterprises	10,948	580	11,528	85	3	88
5. Adventist Health Systems/U.S.	10,715	0	10,715	75	0	75

Source: Modern Healthcare, pp. 65–84, Crain Communications Inc., © May 15, 1984.

lead many nonprofit hospitals to join systems once dominated by for-profit hospitals.

Other market forces that are encouraging the trend toward multi-institutional systems, such as changing clientele, a decline in hospital census, advances in medical technology, reduced government financing, and increased need for management expertise[2] are described below.[3]

The movement of the more affluent population to the suburbs and suburban hospitals has left many urban hospitals with an increasingly elderly, high-risk, sicker, and poor clientele. Because of their high portion of Medicare and Medicaid patients and the increasingly smaller base of private pay and private insurance patients, these hospitals are unable to shift costs of those who cannot pay onto those who can. Because these older hospitals can neither generate nor borrow the capital needed, they often turn to multi-institutional systems or, sometimes, close.

With a decreasing emphasis on inpatient care, hospital occupancy rates have dropped significantly and will continue to do so. Rural hospitals, in particular, continue to lose patients to suburban hospitals and larger teaching institutions, threatening the financial viability of these hospitals and making them prime candidates for multi-institutional system membership.

Because of the high cost of maintaining state-of-the-art technologies and limitations on acquiring them that were set by state regulatory bodies, small and medium-sized hospitals were often unable to obtain many of the more costly new technologies. Too, economies of scale require an increasingly large referral base to support the new technology. The volume required can only be attained through a multi-institutional system.

The decline in philanthrophic giving, especially with the Tax Reform Act of 1986, along with below full cost Medicare and Medicaid reimbursement rates, will make it very difficult for older hospitals to generate enough revenue for their capital needs, especially in view of the unsteadiness of their operating funds. Multi-institutional systems may provide the management expertise and economies of scale to deal with the above pressures assuming that the hospital has a clear direction and understanding of its future role and capital needs priorities. The need for effective institutional planning and management is leading many hospitals to multi-institutional systems for management expertise.

NEW DEVELOPMENTS IN MULTI-INSTITUTIONAL SYSTEMS

In a recent article Tibbits identifies a number of requirements that a new multi-institutional health system must meet to be successful.[3] A successful multi-institutional health system is a system made up not only of a number of hospitals and nursing homes but also of organizations providing outpatient and other services, such as HMOs, preferred provider organizations (PPOs), and home health care organizations (HHCOs). It is an integrated system that provides real returns to its member hospitals in terms of patients, services, and access to a major system of care.

According to Tibbits, to be successful a multi-institutional system or a multihealth corporation must own or operate six to ten hospitals with combined revenues of at least $250 million annually. In addition it must own or control one or more HMOs with at least 100,000 members to provide a solid base of clients. Contracts must also be in place with professional medical corporations to ensure a steady and guaranteed flow of hospital clients. The entire system must be centrally well managed with linked information systems to tie together the decentralized components of its organizations.   The above requirements for success are not at all unusual, except for the stated need of vertical integration. In the past most multi-institutional systems have concentrated on ownership and management of hospitals. The trend in the future will favor vertical integration—rearward through the development or acquisition of HMOs and forward through the acquisition or development of nursing homes and/or home health care organizations.

Many of these local or regional multihealth systems have already joined and in the future more will join health alliances. A health alliance is a voluntary arrangement through which several regional or local multihealth systems band together to take advantage of economies of scale in purchasing, marketing, information systems, financing, and management. Eventually, the local or regional multi-unit health systems will be absorbed by larger nationwide systems. The larger systems will be in a better position to compete in local and regional areas. Even mergers between larger systems will take place. For example, in 1984, Kansas City-based United Healthcare Systems joined Phoenix-based Associated Health Systems to form American Health Care Systems. After the merger, the new conglomerate had 233 member hospitals and revenues of about $5.6 billion. American Health Care became overnight one of the largest nonprofit multi-institutional health systems.

STRATEGIC MANAGEMENT OF MULTI-INSTITUTIONAL SYSTEMS

Strategic management in multi-institutional systems is considerably more complex than in a single hospital system. Multi-institutional systems add one more layer to the hierarchy of the organization.

The logical way to approach strategic management in multi-institutional settings is to use the strategic business unit (SBU) framework discussed in Chapters 10–12. Each self-standing unit in a multi-institutional system then becomes a SBU, and strategic planning then occurs at both the SBU level and at the corporate level. Management and control of the overall organization are handled in a similar fashion.

Whenever organizations grow larger the strategic planning process grows larger also. In addition, the strategic planning process takes longer and usually becomes institutionalized. It typically also extends during the entire year. By a certain time each year, each SBU completes its tentative strategic plan, which it then forwards to the corporate-level planning group. The corporate-level group reviews it and returns it with comments, suggestions, and directions. The SBU then revises its plan and resubmits it. While the SBU is revising its plan and after final plan submission by the SBU, the corporate-level planning team completes its overall corporate plan. A typical planning activity time chart is shown in Figure 19-4. Hence, strategic management for multi-institutional systems becomes a year-round activity and is repeated year after year.

SUMMARY

This industry survey of multi-institutional systems has important implications for the strategic planners of hospitals, multihospital systems, and other

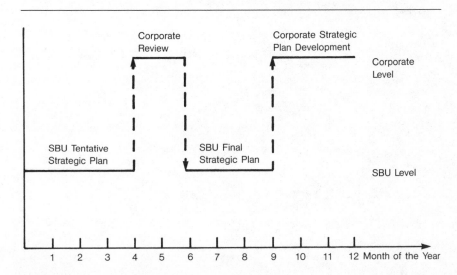

Figure 19-4 Strategic Planning Activity Time Chart

health care institutions. There is an increasing trend toward consolidation and growth in multi-institutional systems.

Although most of the multi-institutional systems are still predominantly operators of hospitals, in the future the revenues from other health-related services will increase. Already, one of the largest multi-institutional systems is the Kaiser Permanente Health Maintenance Organization, a system that derives much of its revenues from hospital operations but is largely a HMO.

Independent hospitals will increasingly have to face the question of continued independence or merger with an existing multi-institutional system. This chapter provides decision-makers with some added information on which to make rational decisions.

NOTES

1. D.E.L. Johnson, "Multi-Unit Providers," *Modern Healthcare,* May 15, 1984, pp. 65–84.

2. W.L. Dowling, "Multi-Hospital Systems Face Growth, Constraints, Unexploited Options," *Health Progress,* April 1983, pp. 48–53.

3. S.J. Tibbits, "Future Belongs to New Multi-Health Corporations—Hospitals Should Join Now," *Modern Healthcare,* September 1984, pp. 203–211.

Chapter 20

Prospective Case Reimbursement and Its Impact on Strategic Planning

20

The federal government's Medicare prospective case reimbursement system, known popularly as the diagnostic-related groups (DRG) reimbursement system, as well as other forms of prospective payment, has required the development of an entirely new set of strategies for hospital management. Hospitals that have been implementing these new strategic plans are the hospitals that will survive and prosper in the years to come. Many hospitals, choosing business as usual, have failed or will fail.

The DRG reimbursement system provides direct financial incentives for hospitals and their staff physicians to handle individual cases in an efficient, low-cost manner. To do so requires more coordination and cooperation among hospital medical staff and management in the management of medical care. It also requires that considerable efforts be put into marketing and evaluation, quality assurance, and consideration of forward and rearward vertical integration.

This chapter explores the impact of prospective payment systems or DRGs on hospitals and how strategic planning steps can be taken to avoid major financial problems.

THE NEED FOR MARKET SEGMENTATION

Consumer market segments have always been defined, analyzed, and related to the types of health services received and to some extent to the age cohort of the population. For instance, acute care services are organized as surgical, pediatric, maternity, and psychiatric care. There also are children's hospital units, adult hospital units, and specific services for older people.

However, the arrival of the DRG brings a need for even sharper segmentation into more defined, sometimes smaller market segments. The senior adult population, for instance, must now be divided into subcategories, typically

259

65-74 years, 75-84 years, and 85 and over.[1] A more refined segmentation on the basis of degree of disability has generated such market segments as ambulatory elderly, homebound elderly, institutionalized elderly, and healthy elderly. Health care and other services that can be provided to these market segments are becoming both more specialized and diverse. Examples are home health care, screening programs, adult day care, nursing home care, acute care, sheltered housing, illness prevention, and health monitoring. Table 20-1 presents a matrix of the degree of health consumer market segmentation that the hospital must consider.

The market segmentation discussed above largely is of the older population. However, in the future, prospective reimbursement for health services will most likely be adopted in some form by Medicaid, commercial health insurance companies, and possibly at some point even by the direct pay patient. New York and other states are moving toward prospective payment reimbursement for nursing homes. Therefore, how much an elective or necessary procedure for any age group will cost must be established before it is performed. This approach—determination of a fee before the service is performed—is common in most other service industries. So why not in health care?

VERTICAL INTEGRATION

Because patients are no longer receiving all of their episodic health care in the acute care setting under DRG reimbursement systems, hospitals need to

Table 20-1 Health Care Market Segmentation Matrix*

	Age Cohorts					
	60–64	65–69	70–74	75–79	80–84	85+
Home health care	– –	–		+	+	+
Day health care	– –	–		+	+	
Nursing home care	– –	– –	–		+	+ +
Screening programs	+ +	+ +	+		–	–
Acute care						
Sheltered housing	– –	–		+	+	
Illness prevention	+ +	+ +	+	+		
Health monitoring	– –	–		+	+ +	+ +

Note: *Indicator in each cell refers to the likelihood that the hospital or health care provider will be able to develop a viable market in the particular market segment to the particular age cohort.

    + + = High Probability
     +   = Probability
          Possibility
     –   = Low probability
    – – = Unlikely

obtain a large share of each patient's nonacute health care as well. This indicates the need for rearward vertical integration through the establishment of ambulatory health care centers, urgent medical care centers, home health care services, and other services that serve those patients who may eventually need hospital care.

Forward vertical integration through the acquisition or development of home health care services, skilled nursing facilities, and health-related facilities provides the hospital with facilities to place the patient following the acute care services performed in the hospital setting. Under DRG reimbursement a fixed sum is paid for hospitalization during a patient's episodic illness or treatment. To provide the medical and health services as economically as possible it is therefore necessary to transfer a patient to a lower-cost environment as soon as possible. The acute care patient should be transferred to a home care or nursing home care environment as soon as medically indicated following the hospital-based care. The hospital that does not own such lower cost health services "loses" the patient to another provider, resulting in significantly lower revenues.

The same relationship holds true for hospital-substitute services such as ambulatory surgery. Under DRGs a significant number of surgeries that were typically done during a 1- or 2-day inpatient stay in a hospital are now *required* to be done on an outpatient, same-day basis. Hospitals not geared up to provide ambulatory surgery are losing a major source of revenue, as well as the inpatient days and complementary ancillary procedure revenues.

DIVERSIFICATION

Vertical integration as a means of system building is a strategy that has the ultimate objective of supporting the parent hospital corporation. In other words, new SBUs, although expected to receive a relatively high rate of return on investment, are primarily focused on system building. Systems are designed to develop complementary rather than competing businesses. Because vertical integration involves the incorporation of new SBUs outside the acute inpatient realm, it is a form of diversification.

However, there is growing consideration of strategies involving true diversification. This next generation of strategies differs primarily in that the SBUs are independent business lines that are not in business to support the hospital but to be successful on their own. It is the profit from their individual success that supports the parent, rather than the systematic development of a flow of patients toward the hospital. Placella discusses two questions that differentiate diversification from system-building/integration strategies: "Is maximizing profits the primary objective? And, is that objective compromised or constrained operationally or geographically?"[2] Can the subsidiary urgent care center establish contracts with otherwise "competing" ancillary services (lab, radiology, etc.)? Can that urgent care center open up shops across the street from the hospital's emergency room? If the answer to these questions is yes, then the strategy is much more closely tied to diversification than to integration. It should be pointed out here that diversification strategies can still be system building. The benefit of system building is, however, secondary to the success of the new venture in terms of its return on investment.

There are several key ingredients to the ultimate success of a diversification strategy. The subsidiaries should be at arm's length from the parent, must have competent profit-oriented management, and should be sufficiently capitalized to allow for success. Diversification is not the right strategy for every hospital; however, it must be considered as an option for its long-term profit potential.

OTHER GROWTH STRATEGIES

A well-thought-out growth strategy is not easily accomplished. It requires considerable additional financial and human resources. Hence, many hospitals cannot afford to engage in expansion of their health services on their own. There are strategies, however, that have minimal capital requirements. The most common strategy is the development of a network of providers who can jointly sponsor the new health services. The network may be formalized in a corporate restructuring and/or merger, or it may be an informal contractual joint venture on a single health service. Hospitals that compete on all other levels have been known to develop a shared service together in order to lower the capital investment required to obtain financing, and fend off competition from nonacute care providers. Many freestanding imaging centers, ambulatory surgery centers, and skilled nursing facilities are the result of hospital joint ventures.

Medical staffs are also involved in joint ventures with hospitals. There are some obvious advantages to hospital-medical staff joint ventures. Physicians are a good source of capital because they are somewhat more investment oriented and have higher incomes than most other professionals. Most have the desire to see "their" hospital succeed, and hospitals depend on the referrals from their community physicians. A joint venture that will be guaranteed by the referrals of the physicians and the support of the hospital is usually already a step ahead of its competition.

A strategy that achieves the same effect as rearward vertical integration yet requires little capital is a major effort to recruit more physicians for active affiliation with the hospital. It has been shown that DRGs have had the effect of creating more competition in the hospital industry as fewer hospital beds will be required. Most hospitals will need to reduce their bed complement, some will close, and others will divide up whatever hospital bed demand remains. Those hospitals that can attract the most effective and productive physician affiliations or who develop ambulatory care or urgent care centers will be the ones that can increase or maintain a necessary market share for economic viability.

Physician bonding is a term that acute care hospitals are beginning to use in their strategic plans to describe the series of strategies that forge stronger linkages between community physicians and the hospital. The overall goal of bonding strategies is to increase physician loyalty and to provide a work environment that will attract new physicians to the hospital staff. There are numerous bonding strategies in use throughout the country. One of the most common is the community physician referral program. Hospitals sponsor and advertise a service whereby the person requiring the services of a physician can call a central phone number and receive the name (or list of names) of a physician who is on the hospital's staff and can meet the person's needs. Although the sophistication of the referral program varies by hospital, all referral services have the same purpose. The physicians have a new source of referral through the hospital, and patients are connected with physicians who will refer them to the hospital when warranted. These programs work best in growth areas where there is a constant influx of new people into the service area. They are surprisingly effective, however, even in established areas because a large proportion of the population does not have a personal physician.

Another form of physician bonding is the hospital-medical staff office linkup. Hospitals are offering their physicians a range of medical practice improvement services, including billing, telephone systems, answering services, information system linkages, and practice management seminars. Many hospitals have hired medical staff sales personnel to work with their physicians and provide products and services to them.

Still another bonding technique, used primarily by major tertiary medical centers, is the referral support service. Physicians are provided with information and liaison services to help facilitate the transfer or referral of their patients needing specialized care. Scheduling, accommodations, transportation, and communication needs of patients are handled through a special hospital office. The referring physician is provided with comprehensive reports on the patient in a timely manner. Patients are no longer lost in the system.

Because many hospitals are already beginning to develop or implement strategies along the lines described above, it is imperative that all hospitals develop strategic plans to respond to the threats they are facing. There has always been a certain measure of competition among hospitals. However, from now on the intensity of competition will increase and only the financially strong hospitals and those hospitals with strong physician affiliations will survive and prosper.

The surviving hospitals of the future will be vastly different from their current counterparts. The surviving hospital will become a vertically integrated and/or diversified health care system. It may have other hospital partners. It will have its own ambulatory care or urgent care centers, and it may even have its own HMO. It will also have its own home health organization, nursing homes, and psychiatric facilities. The health care system of the future will be able to provide the majority of health care needs of the individual and his or her family. A depiction of such a typical integrated system is shown on Figure 20-1.

USE OF EMPTY HOSPITAL SPACE

Of major concern to hospitals faced with lower occupancy rates is the need to develop revenue-generating uses for space once occupied by full hospital beds. A hospital has high fixed capital costs that are not at all affected by bed reductions. Nonproductive use of empty space means that the fixed costs of the hospital must then be allocated to fewer beds, leading to higher costs per case, rather than the lower costs dictated by DRGs. The strategy then must be to find new revenue-producing programs that at least pay for the fixed and variable costs of former bed space.

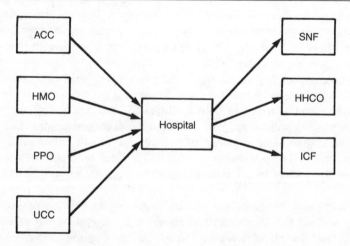

Figure 20-1 Illustration of a Typical Fully Integrated Health Care Organization

The number of new, exciting, and somewhat ingenious uses of hospital space is growing all the time. One use is to provide a new inpatient service. For example, hospitals have turned some of the acute care space into skilled nursing facilities, rehabilitation units, psychiatric units, and alcohol or drug detoxification centers. These new inpatient services, although not at the acute care level, are congruous with the physical resources and professional capabilities of the hospital.

Ambulatory care services are also becoming major sources of revenues to hospitals. Sports medicine and fitness centers, wellness programs, sleep disorder centers, physical rehabilitation and therapy programs, specialty clinics, and diagnostic programs are all providing revenue.

Many hospitals have opened hotel units for families of out-of-town patients or close relatives wishing to stay in proximity to their sick loved ones. Other hospital hotel units are for discharged patients who can receive home health services and rehabilitation programs, as well as the amenities of hotel services. A hospital hotel unit is especially attractive to patients who have no one to care for them at home or whose home atmosphere is not conducive to recuperation. Some hospitals have made several patient rooms into luxury suites, charging additional rates for persons wishing special comforts during their hospital stay.

OUTSIDE CONTRACTING FOR HOSPITAL SERVICES

With the increase in competition will come a search for cost-reduction strategies. Cost reduction achieved through internal and managerial efficiencies should be the first step. The internal hospital structure must be streamlined and revamped to address the revenue restrictions more effectively and to be in a position to move quickly into new areas of opportunity. All hospitals can do a better job of cost control. It is up to management to determine when the return on the cost-cutting effort becomes marginal and is no longer a major budgetary factor.

A very common approach to cost control is outside contracting for hospital services. Many hospitals contract for services that, because of automation, capital investment, or economies of scale, can best be provided through separate contractors that supply the services to more than one hospital. Likely candidates for contracting services are operation of a hospital's computerized information system, its radiology services, and laboratory services. Other candidates for contracting are laundry, meal services, housekeeping, security, and in a few cases even nursing support services. Outpatient surgery, home health care, emergency care, and psychiatric services may also be contracted out.

Outside contractors can usually supply many of the above services at lower cost than the hospital because of their specialization, more intensive use of high-cost capital equipment, expertise, and lower salary costs. The hospital must, however, be on guard that the contractor does not have a monopoly on the service in the area in which the hospital is located. In that case a low contracting price may be charged initially to obtain the contract, but higher charges will quickly follow. At that time it may be difficult for the hospital to return to the old way of doing things itself.

QUALITY ASSURANCE

Of all the potential implications of prospective payment, none has a greater influence on the hospital's future success than does quality of care. It is interesting to note that the quality issue arose more strongly than ever with the simultaneous public interest in medical malpractice cost and the imposition of prospective payment in the early 1980s. Physicians and hospitals were experiencing, on the one hand, pressures to discharge patients earlier and sicker than before and, on the other hand, pressure to prevent incidents that could result in potential lawsuits over poor quality care. Two major results of these conflicting pressures were the further introduction of information systems that monitor hospital usage by physician and/or DRG and far greater sophistication in the discharge planning field to ensure that patients were properly discharged and placed.

Hospitals are not able to trade quality for price. Most physicians and patients expect nothing more than the best possible care. Contracting HMOs and PPOs look to identify only with perceived high-quality institutions. Consumer groups will continue to press for and receive further information on quality outcomes, including mortality rates and nosocomial disease incidence. The popular press will increasingly report on major medical lawsuits or findings of improprieties in local hospitals. The public will be increasingly able to discern the high quality from the average care. Therefore, the successful hospital system of the future will be the one that plans today for the future provision of high-quality care. Major investments must be made in information systems, medical staff and board of trustee education, and proper staffing. The hospital looking for short-term DRG gains through reduction of quality or delaying capital investments will find itself in a poor competitive position over the long run. In addition, the entire organization will be at increasing risk of a major lawsuit that could affect its ability to continue in the health care field.

Quality assurance is the responsibility of the owners and/or board of trustees of a hospital. The medical staff, however, is ultimately the body responsible for implementing quality care. Therefore, the quality assurance program must be a strong partnership between the board and medical staff, with a total commitment on both ends. Physician credentialing should be in place to ensure that aggressive physician recruitment programs recruit only qualified practitioners. Utilization review must counteract the tendency to fill beds unnecessarily. Incident reporting must be effectively monitored through an organized risk management program. These investments will lead to far greater long-run returns than any new program or service.

SUMMARY

This chapter discussed the structural changes that are and will be taking place because of the implementation of the DRG system, first for Medicare patients and eventually for Medicaid patients and the general population now covered by health insurance plans, HMOs, and private pay.

DRG implementation has and will provide considerable impetus to forward vertical integration, that is, hospital ownership or involvement in home health care, nursing homes, and other posthospital programs. It will stimulate rearward vertical integration through the development of improved medical staff relations, ambulatory care, and/or urgent care centers. Rearward vertical integration is necessary in order to increase a hospital's market share so it can utilize its resources more efficiently and effectively. Diversification should be considered as an option as well. With many hospitals vying for the same market, unprepared hospitals will lose market share and as a result encounter financial difficulties and possible financial collapse.

Hospitals need to develop strategic plans that reflect the above scenario and react to it to ensure survival. In developing these strategic plans hospitals must keep in mind the basics of quality assurance and medical staff bonding. The restructuring of the hospital from an acute care hospital to a comprehensive health care institution requires the cooperation and support of all levels of management, medical staff, and the board of trustees.

NOTES

1. Alan M. Zuckerman, "The Impact of DRG Reimbursement on Strategic Planning," *ACHA/ Journal* 29, no. 4, (July/August 1984): 40–49

2. Louis E. Placella, "Choosing a Growth Strategy: Diversification versus Vertical Integration," *Trustee*, November, 1986, 12–19.

Chapter 21

Seizing the
Competitive Initiative

HIGHLIGHTS

- Influencing Forces
- How To Compete
- Knowing Where You Are
- Individual and Collective Goals
- Ten Pitfalls
- Communication

21

This chapter addresses strategic planning, about what we at Warner-Lambert call "seizing the competitive initiative." It is not going to teach you how to do strategic planning. Instead it provides a perspective on the kind of thinking involved in strategic planning as we at Warner-Lambert do it. The chapter also gives you a sense of the pitfalls that await you when you implement any strategic plan. I know these pitfalls well, since I have been involved in strategic planning at Warner-Lambert from the day 6 years ago when we began to formally address the subject. I have the bruises that come from falling into some of the pitfalls I will describe, and I hope I have the alertness that comes from avoiding some of the others.

Ten years ago—even 5 years—the idea that hospitals and other health care institutions might actually think about, worry about, and participate in competition with other hospitals and health care institutions would have been called a fantasy by some, a nightmare by others. It is no longer either; it is a reality.

INFLUENCING FORCES

Indeed, that strategic planning and competition are facts of life and survival is a tribute to several issues that are affecting health care institutions in this country. I use the word "tribute" in the older sense of the word—an acknowledgment of the power of an external force.

Source: Reprinted from "Seizing the Competitive Initiative: Strategic Planning in the Health Care Field" by M.R. Goodes, *Hospital & Health Services Administration*, Vol. 29, No. 4, pp. 30–39, with permission of the Foundation of the American College of Healthcare Executives, © 1984.

What are those forces, those issues? A brief list of the most important will be as well known to you as they are to me.

One, the soaring cost of health care in this country. In 1982, Americans spent more than \$322 billion on health care—10.5 percent of the gross national product. And, of direct concern to you here, the largest part of that health care cost was the amount spent in the nation's hospitals—\$136 billion, excluding physicians' services.

These staggering figures alone have resulted in a major push by politicians, by business leaders, and by consumers for cost containment all along the line, spawning all those bumps in the night that keep us all awake: DRGs, HMOs, prospective payment programs, and so on.

Two, an increasing oversupply of physicians. There are now nearly 500,000 physicians in the United States, and the medical schools are graduating nearly 16,000 new ones every year.

An important consequence of that oversupply is that it has spawned new competitors out of the ranks of those who were traditionally an integral part of the hospital system. Those who once were solely your partners are now potentially and actually your competitors.

Three, a national demand for increasing quality of health care. No one can possibly object to increasing quality of anything, much less to increasing quality in health care. But this demand, in many cases, runs counter to the cost-containment drive.

Four, internal cost pressure, especially in the labor market. While the thrust of cost containment has been largely focused on supplies, devices, and prescriptions, these represent only 17 percent of the typical hospital costs. Other costs are harder to reduce, even though they are a more important source of internal and external discontent.

Five, regulatory issues. Deregulation may still be a trend in political and national economic life, but I strongly suspect we will never see it in our fields. Instead, new regulations like certificates of need and third party payments will continue to be piled on top of the regulatory issues that we all face stemming from OSHA and HHA.

Six, last, and not least, there are the new forms of competition: the growing for-profit hospital corporations, hospices, home health care, etc.

HOW TO COMPETE

What you are faced with, in business terms, are rising costs, rising consumer expectations, new forms of government regulation, new kinds of competition, labor problems, and product price limitations. It is no longer a question of whether a hospital should compete—only a question of how to compete, and how to compete in such a way to ensure your institution's survival and continued effectiveness.

The question, then, is "how to compete in the marketplace?" For us at Warner-Lambert, the essence of strategic planning is in those words: "how," "compete," and "marketplace." Those three words, and what they represent, must be analyzed, planned for, and pursued at two different levels: at the level of each strategic business unit and at the aggregate level, which is the level of the institution as a whole.

The planning process for us is keyed off by two of these words—compete and marketplace—and it begins with a careful, thoughtful analysis of each of our strategic business units in relation to each of their competitors. We look at the strengths of each unit—whether that strength is in manufacturing cost or productivity, in distribution, in product quality or cost, in management skills, and on and on—because each of those strengths is, by definition, a competitor's weakness.

Similarly, we look at the weaknesses of each unit—again, no matter where in the raw-material-to-customer-pocket process—because each of those weaknesses is a competitor's strength.

Then we look at the marketplace for each of those units. Who are those customers? How many of them does each unit have? What percentage of the total possible does each unit have? Why are the customers buying or not buying? Which customers do we want to have—because, after all, you can not have them all; it is not possible in any real world.

Then with all this information, each business unit knows where it is now.

KNOWING WHERE YOU ARE

Some may say that knowing where you are now is not important. After all, strategic planning and thinking is figuring out where you want to be at some point in the future. What good is knowing where you are now, particularly since "now" immediately recedes into the past, and all you really ever find out is where you were when?

But knowing where you are is important, even if that "now"is some recent past because you cannot devise a road map to a future goal unless you know where you are starting from.

Back to the planning process. With this information about now, each unit then decides where it wants to be at some definite point in the future. To do that, it must also decide where it can seize the competitive initiative, where it can gain advantages that its competitors cannot, at least not immediately. It can do that in a number of ways, two of which are most important to you. First, each business unit segments its market. It can decide to take that universe of actual and potential consumers and go after a particular segment of that group. It can, like Mercedes, decide it will go after only the affluent and would-be affluent market. Or it can, like McDonald's, go after the lower and lower-middle income market. There is profit in both, but each means a different kind of product or service and a different kind of marketing.

Second, each business unit tailors its offer or, in other words, produces and markets its product with a specifically designed appeal. Mercedes, for example, does not really compete with Ford or Chrysler. It competes with European vacations and backyard swimming pools.

But each business unit does all this differentiation and tailoring in the light where it wants to be and where its competitors are likely to want to be.

INDIVIDUAL AND COLLECTIVE GOALS

And when all this information is gathered, the whole process is repeated for the company as a whole. In that way, the company can decide whether it wants to invest heavily in one business unit because its prospects for growth or profitability or both are bright or whether it wants to get out of another business unit because there is little likelihood of that unit ever seizing a significant competitive initiative.

After all this information is gathered for each unit and for the aggregate corporation, and all the analysis is completed, and everyone has set individual and collective goals—only then is the third word of the three key words addressed—the "how." And that how is the action plan, both individual and corporate, for achieving those goals.

The whole process takes time and a lot of energy, some late nights, and some quiet desperation. But, in essence, it is simple enough. There are lots of ways of thinking about the process, lots of "x" and "y" axes on graph paper, lots of simple and complicated formulas. But, in essence, it involves the kind of clear, objective, hard-headed, logical thinking that most of us find inordinately difficult, especially when what we are talking about involves our lives.

In some ways, the strategic planning process up to this point is the easy part. The pitfalls, the real dangers, lie beyond.

Where are they? They lie on the difficult road called "implementation." After all, if you and your family decide to drive to San Francisco from Hartford, getting out the road maps, planning the route, and taking the car to the garage for a tune-up is time-consuming, may involve a number of arguments, and costs money. But the problems only begin when you pack up the car and leave the driveway.

TEN PITFALLS

The same is true for strategic planning. From my own experience, I have identified ten key pitfalls you must watch for and avoid at all costs.

Pitfall One, or "You cannot drive a car without a driver." No plan, and no planning process, can work unless the concept of strategic planning has complete commitment from the top. Such commitment is not all you need, but it is a sine qua non. As I am sure you have all experienced in one part of your life or another, there is nothing an organization so quickly senses and reacts to as the intimation from its leaders that something or other is really not to be taken seriously.

And words of commitment are never enough. Most organizations have been through a variety of fads, schemes, or plans that really did not have to be paid attention to. After all, there is a job to be done, a service to be delivered, a product to be produced, and if "the old man" really does not care, I certainly do not.

No, that commitment has to mean that top managers must take an active part, must be seen to take time, to expend energy, and to visibly expect others to follow their example. At Warner-Lambert, our CEO, Ward Hagan, has been so committed from the very beginning. Sure, we have made considerable use of outside consultants for a variety of tasks. But, even from the beginning, executives and top-level management were deeply involved in the planning process. And, in the end, the strategic planning was their strategic planning.

Pitfall Two, or "You can not start out unless everyone is in the car." The bottom-up planning process that I have described from my Warner-Lambert experience is designed to avoid this pitfall. By working this way, you get the very people who are responsible for carrying out the plan involved in formulating it. It becomes their plan, too, and it is very difficult to avoid responsibility and accountability for achieving goals if you are the one who set the goals and laid out the way you were going to achieve the goals. If you fail, you either have to admit that you failed or that you were a bad planner—and neither admission tends to do much for your career.

So, with commitment from the top and commitment from the bottom, you can be sure you and your family can get on the road. Or can you?

There is always the dreaded Pitfall Three or, "The plan as an end in itself." Strategic planning is such a buzzword that far too many companies feel that just having a plan is enough. This is a pitfall most easily encountered when the plan is drawn up by outsiders, but even companies that draw up their own are susceptible. It just looks good, all bound up with a slick cover on it and lots of tabs and a table of contents. And it fits so nicely into the filing cabinet or the desk drawer!

But a strategic plan without an action plan is no plan at all. It is merely a collective wish list, full of pious hopes and resolves. And the action plan itself contains another pitfall.

Pitfall Four, or "The road without milestones." The action plan that is the culmination of a strategic plan must have points at which progress toward the agreed-upon goals is checked and measured. How else can you tell how you are doing and what kind of progress you're making? How else can you judge the quality of your managers and the quality of your plan?

And checkpoints involve a regular, periodic review of each business unit and the aggregate whole. If this is beginning to sound like strategic planning and seizing the strategic initiative is a never-ending process, that is what it is supposed to sound like. In fact, the ultimate goal of all strategic planning is to inculcate it so deeply into everyone's mind that it becomes strategic thinking. And that's when you know that you are on your way to real success.

Unless, of course, you fall prey to Pitfall Five.

Pitfall Five is when you allow assumptions to become facts. All planning involves a great number of assumptions. You assume the marketplace will look a certain way. You assume the technology will develop in a particular direction. You assume that costs will continue to rise in a specific curve. You assume and you assume.

But assumptions are not facts. The future never contains facts. And for that reason, you must constantly remind yourself that those assumptions are just that—assumptions. You must keep testing and retesting those assumptions, for if anyone of them turns out to be wrong, then your plan must change. If you have assumed that, by now, Nebraska must have completed that part of the interstate and that, by now, surely the road crews in Pennsylvania will have cleared that landslide—but the rocks are still covering the roadside of Pittsburgh and the detour signs outside Lincoln point to a dirt road—you have just got to change your plans. Or sit in your car and watch the kids kill each other in the back seat.

Checking your assumptions also means keeping flexible. New developments occur all the time. After all, DRGs came on far more quickly and in a different form than anyone really expected. So, as I discuss a bit later, your information systems are as much a part of competing and of seizing the competitive initiative as is cost containment.

Which brings us to the next problem to watch out for.

Pitfall Six, or "You can't drive the car in five different directions at once." You can't drive it simultaneously in two different directions. In reviewing the plan, and in checking progress along the way, keep in mind the need for internal consistency in planning and implementation. The larger the organization, and the more independent and powerful the unit and division managers, the easier it is for parts of the organization to be pulling in different, even contrary directions. If you are not careful, someone may be out there buying up a steel mill because the price is so good when everyone else is trying to move the company into consumer food products. Or someone buys the tenth CAT scanner in town because he can not stand being the only department chief without one and his research depends on it.

And do not forget Pitfall Seven, or "Confusing hopes with objectives." Survival or profitability are not objectives—they are hopes or aspirations. An objective is measurable, observable, and, if chosen correctly, achievable. Attaining a 40 percent share of the adult popsicle market is an objective. Attaining a 12 percent return on equity is an objective. Hiring the best automobile engine designer in the country is an objective. Having dinner at the Top of the Mark and looking out into San Francisco Bay is an objective.

Then there is Pitfall Eight, or "You can not drive to San Francisco in one day, and you can not drive to London at all." There is always real danger in planning of encouraging or forcing people into unrealistic goals. Overexpectation or overpromising will ruin a plan—and demoralize the people without whom the plan is just a lot of processed trees—and just when all your competitors are trying to seize that initiative, too. Any good plan will have goals that will make people stretch to achieve them, that will make them try harder and smarter than they did last year. But "stretch" goals must be attainable ones.

There are just two pitfalls left to go.

Pitfall Nine, or "When you give out the rewards, make sure you know what the rewards are for." Nothing tells people in an organization what is expected of them more surely and more quickly than the reward system—and I do not care whether those rewards are lollipops, wall plaques, or money. Your organization must have rewards for people achieving their goals, but there is a trap here. If the only rewards are given for meeting short-term goals—say, driving 500 miles a day—you must also have some system of rewards for long-term thinking and long-term goals. After all, anyone can continue to drive 500 miles a day endlessly—and drive those 500 miles in a continuous circle.

A long-term strategic plan can and must consist of a series of short-term goals. But a series of short-term goals, put together by people who are only encouraged to think in the short term, does not necessarily add up to a long-term plan. And only long-term thinking, planning, and action will ensure survival—as the American automobile industry has found out after a great deal of pain.

And that inevitably brings us to the last pitfall.

Pitfall Ten, or "You cannot drive the car all by yourself." Everyone must learn to drive. The ultimate point of strategic planning is to make everyone a strategic thinker and strategic manager. Keeping strategic planning as an isolated staff function will ultimately lead to the disappearance of strategic planning as an important part of organizational life.

COMMUNICATION

As mentioned earlier, the real aim of planning is to embed it into the way people think every day and into the way they act every day. That means lots of communication in all directions—top-down, bottom-up, and sideways. Communication is not only the way to keep track of how things are going. It is also the only way to transmit information. Information gathering is not only important to the construction of the plan, it is also critical to the implementation of the plan. Indeed, planning and checking, explaining and revising, checking up and communicating back—these are all different ways of saying "information systems." In a real sense, your whole organization is an information system waiting to be tapped. And tap it you must, because planning is not only an unceasing process. It is, when done well, a constantly communicated and informed one.

Those are the ten most dangerous pitfalls on the way to successfully seizing the competitive initiative. After listening to my description, many of you may be anxious about this process. Others may be angry that such steps are necessary. Still others may be eager to get out there and compete. I can understand all those emotions, but it is this last group who is right. Rather than being something scary or irritating, competition and acting to seize the competitive advantage will work for you as it has worked for all the other industries in this country. It will prove to be the best thing that has happpened to you, to your physicians and nurses, to your staff—and to health care in America. Competition really does work to improve cost, quality, and service. I have seen it happen at Warner-Lambert. I promise that you will see it happen, too.

Chapter 22

The Link between Strategic Planning and Implementation

22

Much of the dissatisfaction with strategic planning in recent years can be traced to the unsatisfactory implementation of strategic plans. There are of course many plausible reasons for the poor implementation performance, and some of these are addressed in this chapter.

The first reason is the unacknowledged link between strategic plan development and plan implementation. Strategic plans developed by outside consultants or internal strategic planning staffs that are then handed down or imposed on line management are especially bound to lack credibility. They are perceived in many cases as a challenge to line management not to perform. They are frequently viewed as outside interference, and by not executing these plans satisfactorily management is expressing its dissatisfaction with having been excluded from the strategic planning process. The above scenario may be a bit extreme, but it is considered one of the main reasons for poor strategic plan implementation.

How can this problem be avoided? Clearly, one way is to involve line management in the strategic plan development process. This can be costly because it takes line management staff away from solving their current problems, and it may even impose additional work on them. However, it is imperative that the management groups who are expected to implement whatever changes are embedded in the strategic plan are active participants in it and approve the strategic plan. This does not imply that each line manager must partake in all aspects of strategic planning, but he or she must certainly be actively involved in that aspect of the planning process that is relevant to him or her.

Participation in the strategic planning process by itself is, however, not enough. Too, all levels of management must think strategically. Strategic thinking is constantly thinking in terms of where the organization is and should be heading. Worrying in a positive way may even be a more proper term for explaining what is strategic thinking.

It is not easy to convince or train management to think strategically. It is a form of management culture for which management should be trained, and the training process should be made part of the regular management development activities of the organization. If strategic thinking is not actively cultivated, there will be a tendency for line management staff to concentrate their energies solely on current problems.

This chapter also presents six common barriers to strategy implementation and discusses how strategy, especially strategy implementation, can be linked to performance evaluation. Although good performance measures usually exist for current performance, relatively poor or no performance measures exist for strategy implementation performance. The last section addresses this problem and makes some suggestions for improvement.

STRATEGIC THINKING AND STRATEGY IMPLEMENTATION

Strategic planning is only one part of strategic management. It is necessary but not sufficient for strategic management to succeed. Strategic management comprises a range of activities from strategic planning to strategy implementation.

Numerous articles have been written in recent years criticizing strategic planning because of its inability to effect strategic change. A strategic plan by itself is of course only a document that is worthless if it is not implemented. The criticism of strategic planning is thus essentially directed at strategy implementation or the lack thereof.

Michael Porter points out that one of the reasons for lack of strategy implementation is the lack of strategic thinking on the part of management.[1] Yet, the need for strategic thinking has never been greater. Unless strategic thinking is part of the corporate culture, it rarely occurs spontaneously. Day-to-day operating problems tend to crowd out any opportunities for strategic thinking by management, that is, when management constantly thinks in terms of future implications of what it is doing now. It is true that the formal strategic planning process creates opportunities for management to participate in brainstorming and strategic thinking. However, strategic thinking needs to be much more pervasive over time, and it needs to involve more than just the top management group.

Strategic thinking as a critical part of management, and not just top management, has the potential to create an environment in which strategy implementation is viewed as a direct extension of strategic thinking and strategy plan formulation. If all levels of management think strategically and if the strategic plan has been developed with full participation by all levels of management, then those managers who are responsible for implementing their parts of the strategic plan will do so willingly and enthusiastically. In contrast, if a strategic plan is imposed from above—that is, if top management develops the strategic plan without consultation and input from lower levels of management—then strategy implementation can be expected to be difficult. Lower-level management will view the implementation of the strategic plan as something in which they have no part. Consequently, they will show little enthusiasm to assist in implementation of the strategic plan.

Without strategic thinking there is a tendency to concentrate solely on current problems and ignore the larger long-term problems and directions in which the organization should be directed and guided. Strategic thinking requires strong top managment leadership. Top management must also constantly remind the lower and middle levels of management of the importance of strategic thinking. This can be done through workshops, seminars, retreats or at regular management meetings. Without constant reminding that management should think strategically, there is a tendency to fall in the trap of concentrating solely on current problems.

SIX BARRIERS TO STRATEGY IMPLEMENTATION

Implementation difficulties frequently have deeper roots than one would expect. As Gray points out, implementation difficulties frequently can be attributed to the following preimplementation factors:[2]

1. poor preparation of line managers
2. faulty definition of business units
3. vaguely formulated goals
4. inadequate information bases for action planning
5. badly handled reviews of business unit plans
6. inadequate linkage of strategic planning with other control systems

It is now widely accepted that strategic planning is a line management function in which staff specialists play a supporting role. Unfortunately, the staff specialist frequently ends up playing the leading role, and line managers become merely information contributors to the strategic plan. It is very important that line managers view the strategic plan as their plan and that they feel responsible for its implementation. Therefore, it is desirable to require line management to sign off on the strategic plan documents. The sign-off process should be more than just a formality. It should occur following document review sessions in which line managers can modify the document as a group. In other words, the strategic plan preparation process becomes a review process, followed by a consensus agreement on the final document. Although this process is time consuming it will pay for itself in successful implementation results.

Defining the business unit is critical in strategic plan formulation. Whether the SBU is a multibillion dollar unit or a small division in a corporation, it is important that clear lines of unit and responsibility demarcation are drawn. Line managers must be clear about their responsibilities.

Poorly formulated goals can also be hazards that impede implementation. Goals and objectives should be specific and tied to action plans. Well-formulated goals and objectives, which can also serve as performance indicators, guide line managers in performing actions for which they are responsible.

Action plans should not only be specific and detailed but they should also be tied to goals and objectives. In other words a well-developed strategic plan not only sets goals and objectives by consensus but also develops agreed-upon action plans to implement the strategy that will satisfy the goals and the objectives. Action plans should also be set in a proper time framework. Management can thus determine at any one time during the strategic plan implementation phase how much has been accomplished and how much still needs to be completed.

A poor review of the plans of a business unit is largely a communication problem. If top management does not fully understand the business unit plans then these plans should be returned to the business unit for clarification. In turn each business unit is entitled to a thorough and critical review of its submitted plan by top management. The danger in this process is the tendency to do top-down planning. That is, the business unit line managers may not view the plan as their own if top management makes too many changes in the plan. Yet, top management must ensure that the business unit plan fits in with the corporate strategic direction. If conflicts arise, it is very important that these conflicts be straightened out without alienating line management of the business unit.

Because strategic planning in many corporations is considered a relatively new and intermittent activity, the linkage of strategic planning with older and existing control systems usually has not been established. This lack can be a major hindrance to implementation. For instance, if a line manager's performance is evaluated on the basis of an existing production, financial, or quality control system, he or she will pay more attention to those controls than to goals and objectives specified in a strategic plan. Hence, it is of utmost importance that line management be aware that their evaluation is based as much on strategy implementation as it is on performing satisfactorily in respect to existing control systems. Ideally, of course, the goals and objectives specified in the strategic plan should become part of the existing control systems. In many instances this is feasible, but in many others it is not.

LINKING STRATEGY IMPLEMENTATION AND PERFORMANCE EVALUATION

How can managers be motivated to achieve the goals and objectives embedded in the strategic plan? Migliore addresses this issue and proposes that managers be evaluated on the basis of five to ten key performance objectives and ten specific criteria.[3]

The five to ten key performance criteria are common quantitative specific performance factors concerning budget, production output, quality level, sales level, etc. The ten specific criteria are more qualitative:

1. use of long-range planning
2. developing people
3. contribution to morale
4. communication
5. creativity
6. emotional stability
7. job knowledge
8. what kind of leader
9. problem solver
10. public image/social responsibility

A similar rating scale could be developed for the quantitative performance factors and for the qualitative evaluation criteria. Migliore suggests a five-level scale consisting of excellent, above average, average, below average, and poor. Each of the levels could then be given a quantitative score, such as 5 for excellent, 4 for above average, etc. A weighting scheme could then be used for weighting the performance factors one way and the evaluation criteria another way. Thus, a single quantitative evaluation value could be derived that would enable management to compare the members of the management group. The evaluation method could of course also be used without rating and weighting. Whatever approach is used depends on management's preference.

The purpose of using the above evaluation scheme is to include factors that explicitly measure a manager's level of participation in strategic thinking, strategic planning, and strategy implementation. The ten evaluation criteria may need to be modified to do so. However, they form the basis or a model from which a reasonable management evaluation tool can be developed.

FUTURE NEEDS AND DIRECTIONS

Strategic management is a relatively young discipline and is still evolving. In the health care environment it is especially young, and therefore it is very difficult to determine what impact it will have in the health care environment in the future.

To be successful, strategic management must be able to foster strategic thinking on the part of all levels of management and also on other spheres of influence, such as affiliated physicians and board members. Strategic thinking requires that people are able to identify a path from where the organization is now to where it will go into the future. Strategic thinking also requires that management think and identify more with the entire organization as opposed to identifying with their own area of interest and expertise. The challenge of top management will therefore be to motivate the organization to muster its managerial and other influential sources to think strategically and in a consensus, or at least near-consensus fashion, about the direction in which the organization should move.

Strategic thinking by itself is, of course, not sufficient to move an organization in the proper direction. The proper strategy still needs to emanate from the strategic thinking process. However, strategic thinking is a necessary condition. Organizations that are able to marshal their leadership groups to think strategically will therefore be in a much better position than organizations that are run autocratically with top-down management and top-down strategic management.

Hence, strategic management will evolve into a consensus-building and participative-style organization building movement. This does not preclude continuation of the strategic plan development process. The planning documents still need to be prepared. However, more effort will go into developing strategic plans that have strong support from all levels of management and also from sources external to management, such as affiliated physicians and board members.

SUMMARY

The linkage between strategic planning, strategic thinking, and strategy implementation was the topic of this chapter. Probably the most important way to ensure satisfactory implementation of a strategic plan is to have line management participate and agree by consensus to those aspects of the strategic plan for which they are responsible. Most strategic plans are prepared by outside or staff planning specialists with no or minimal input from line management. Under those conditions strategy implementation will be difficult, if not impossible. As a result many organizations that proceeded this way have become disappointed and disillusioned with the strategic planning process.

Strategic thinking does not come naturally. It must be reinforced through workshops, management development, and other types of management training sessions. Because strategy implementation activities are not routine or repetitive the means of evaluating them are not always in place. As a result management performance in respect to strategy implementation is frequently overlooked. In the future, more attention will likely be paid to strategic thinking and to consensus building. Both are required to ensure satisfactory implementation of developed strategic plans.

NOTES

1. M.E. Porter, "The State of Strategic Thinking," *The Economist* 303, no. 7499 (May 23, 1987): 17–22.

2. D.H. Gray, "Uses and Misuses of Strategic Planning," *Harvard Business Review,* January–February, 1986, 15–28.

3. R.H. Migliore, "Linking Strategy, Performance, and Pay," *The Journal of Business Strategy* 3, no. 1 (Summer 1982): 10–18.

Index

Public response, environmental
analysis, 60

Q

Quick ratio, 112

R

Rating scales, competitive analysis,
73, 74
Ratios
application of
financial viability of hospital
example, 119–122
time-series analysis, 115–116
See also Financial/operating ratios.
Rearward vertical integration, 103–104
Referral support service, physician
bonding, 263
Regulatory changes, environmental
analysis, 60, 61
Reorganization, 106–108, 127
foundation model, 107–108
models for
basic model, 106–107
strong hospital model, 107
success/failure factors, 106
Representative participation, 7
Retrospective planning, 8
Return-on-assets ratio, 113
Return-on-equity ratio, 113
Return-on-revenue ratio, 113

S

Service area
analysis of, as step in planning, 35–36
geographic area, 71–72
Wheatfield Hospital example
competition, 50
demographics, 46–47, 48–49

Service area attractiveness
mission department business
strength matrix
illustrations of, 188–191, 200–205
scale used, 185–187
SBU business strength matrix,
155–159
illustrations of, 157–159, 167–170
scale used, 155–156
Service departments (SD)
definition of, 99
examples of, 99
in planning process, 99–100
Social changes, environmental
analysis, 60
Solo physician's office, 211
Strategic business units (SBU)
definition of, 98
description of, 97–98
matrix analysis
growth share matrix, 147–151
service area attractiveness, SBU
business strength matrix,
155–159
Strategic implementation
barriers to, 283–284
and performance evaluation, 285
poor implementation, reasons for, 281
strategic thinking and, 282–283
Strategic management
ambulatory health care centers,
211–218
health maintenance organizations
(HMOs), 221–230
home health care, 233–241
multi-institutional systems, 254–255
See also specific topics
Strategic planning
ambulatory health care centers,
217–218
as collaborative process, 101
corporate planning, 101
generic strategies, 102–103
horizontal integration, 105–106
reorganization, 106–108
vertical integration, 103–104